THE
"ABORTION PILL"

RU-486 · A Woman's Choice

Etienne-Emile Baulieu
with Mort Rosenblum

SIMON & SCHUSTER

New York   London   Toronto   Sydney   Tokyo   Singapore

SIMON & SCHUSTER

Simon & Schuster Building
Rockefeller Center
1230 Avenue of the Americas
New York, New York 10020

Designed by Laurie Jewell
Manufactured in the United States of America

1   3   5   7   9   10   8   6   4   2

Library of Congress Cataloging-
in-Publication Data

Baulieu, Etienne-Emile.
[Génération pilule. English]
The abortion pill : RU-486, a woman's choice / Etienne-Emile
Baulieu with Mort Rosenblum.
p. cm.
Translation of: Génération pilule.
Includes index.
1. Mifepristone—Research—History. 2. Abortion—Moral and
ethical aspects. I. Rosenblum, Mort. II. Title.
[DNLM: 1. Mifepristone—history—France. 2. Mifepristone—
personal narratives. QV 11 B346g]
RG137.6.M53B3813 1991
613.9′432—dc20
DNLM/DLC
for Library of Congress   91-5054
                                                       CIP

ISBN: 0-671-73816-X

"Science has an essential virtue; it respects what is."
PRIMO LEVI

"Woman is the future of man."
LOUIS ARAGON

"[Margaret Sanger] launched a movement that is obeying a higher law to preserve human life under human conditions."
MARTIN LUTHER KING

CONTENTS

Chapter One

THE
UNPREGNANCY
PILL

THE PRIMORDIAL human race, three hundred million sperm in pursuit of an egg, is still mysterious. Up close, this microscopic contest is as dramatic and inevitable as the movement of planets. When a sperm pierces the egg, it resembles a twisting tornado burrowing into a moon's surface. Symbolically, this marks a new life. Scientifically, it is the beginning of the beginning.

From ovulation to the last pains of labor, the process is a seamless continuum. Each month, an egg, crowned by a halo of nutrient cells called the corona radiata, descends from the ovary to the fallopian tube. The cervix and uterus secrete fluids, and tiny channels no wider than a hair form within the cervical mucus. These are the pathways sought by sperm.

Sperm can travel six inches in a few hours, each sperm propelled by a "tail," the flagellum, and driven by an energy pack, the mitochondria. Many never penetrate the uterus. Some probe the wrong fallopian tube. Others die on the way. Perhaps two hundred eventually approach the egg.

The tiny horde of sperm batters the egg. No sperm can penetrate until its acrosome opens; this sac of enzymes helps the head work its way past nutrient cells and through the egg's pliable shell, the zona pellucida. After several hours of probing, the acrosome wears thin, and the egg is vulnerable. A single sperm, no bigger than one twentieth of a millimeter, fuses with the egg's inner membrane. Then it burrows into the cell plasma to fertilize the egg.

To some, a new person joins the world at fertilization. This romantic notion captivates us all: the union of sperm and egg like the act of love which made it possible. But we scientists know that little has occurred at this point: as the race finishes, an obstacle course begins.

Freed of its driving tail, the sperm head is a mass of genes which merge not instantaneously but over a period of many hours, with the egg's corresponding genes. Each sperm is different. One might carry half the makings of a Mozart; the next, a mutant. The outcome depends on which gets there first.

The egg is also unique, different from others that evolved in the ovary but were not released. The sperm and egg form twenty-two pairs of chromosomes plus a twenty-third, an X of maternal origin and another X (to form a female) or a Y (specifying a male) from the sperm. Genes of both mother and father have divided in a process called meiosis to form the germ cells, egg and sperm. These halves mix and match with such complexity that possible combinations among the one hundred thousand genes in each chromosome can total 10^{2000}. The atoms in the universe, as we know it, add up to a far smaller number.

Less than two days after intercourse, genetic lines are drawn in the fertilized egg, or zygote. Fewer than half of all zygotes will survive. Most pass out of the body, and no pregnancy occurs. Some divide, thus preparing for the development of more than one person. Others grow into tumors, meaning no human being will develop. But each now contains the potential makings of a child. Whether that child would be capable of setting an Olympic record or is fated to suffer a congenital deformity, the die has been cast.

Events happen quickly. The zygote is swept down the fallopian tube toward the uterus by waves of microscopic hairs called cilia. Contractions help to squeeze it along. The trip takes three days, during which the zygote develops into a morula (Latin for "mulberry") with sixteen cells. When the morula approaches the uterus, it divides into about a hundred cells, the size of a pinhead. It is now a primitive embryo, a blastocyst.

The blastocyst eases into the womb and, for a few days, bumps about like a tiny balloon. Then it sheds its protective zona pellucida and implants itself, usually toward the top of the uterus. As the little module lands, it lowers tiny legs made of sugar molecules. These link up with similar molecules in the uterine wall to hold the blastocyst in place. Progesterone has prepared the way. The Latin-derived name of this steroid hormone, made from cholesterol, suggests its crucial role in pregnancy: *pro* (for) and *gestare* (to carry). It is secreted by the corpus luteum, made of ovarian cells produced during ovulation.

Before implantation, progesterone thickens the uterine lining, the endometrium, making it hospitable. Once the blastocyst attaches itself, it makes a second hormone, human chorionic gonadotropin (hCG), which enters the woman's bloodstream and energizes the corpus luteum. As a result, more progesterone flows, which sends a message to the brain to suppress the next ovulation. Later, as the embryo develops into a fetus, its placenta secretes yet more progesterone. This calms uterine contractions, protecting the embryo from being dislodged.

On the fourteenth day or so after fertilization, a tiny furrow in the blastocyst signals that it is no longer capable of splitting into twins. This is the "primitive streak," and now the process of producing a child begins in earnest.

Few clues have yet reached the mother about the drama taking place in her deepest recesses. Some women say they know instinctively. Most notice only that their period is late, and without a hormonal test they are not sure why. In biological terms, the father has done his part. The process is within the mother, and it is she who must decide what to do.

The moral dilemmas, like the physiological options, begin at this stage. The essence of love, the comfort of family, the survival of the human race itself all figure in the miracle of childbearing. Some religions hold this to be sacred. Philosophy and literature ponder its deeper meanings. There is little in this world to match the light in a woman's eyes when she learns what is taking place and is happy about it.

But human life is as complex as the process that conceives it. In a world approaching a population of six billion, with poverty and sickness and sexual assault, this blessed event may well be cursed. No one can decide that for a woman, but science can help her act on her decision. The goal of providing women with new options has inspired my research for over twenty years.

The embryo develops swiftly. By the fifth week after fertilization, it is crescent-shaped, a centimeter long. The rudimentary human beginning takes a strange animal form. A backbone curves from the first trace of a brain to a taillike protrusion. The embryonic heart pumps blood to the liver. In three more weeks, although it weighs less than an ounce and measures four centimeters, all the organs of a fully grown human are in place. At twelve weeks, it can be called a fetus.

Although the brain is far from developed at this point, the fetus moves a little and responds to stimuli in the mother as its nerve fibers connect. After four months, it seems to start testing its body systems. There is "quickening," an old term for the first time a mother feels movement inside of her. At seven months, the fetus can open its eyes as if to look for a way out. At nine months, it finds one.

A bad shock can dislodge an embryo or a fetus from the womb. Often, an unwilling mother's only recourse is to hope this happens. Ancient civilizations concocted gruesome options; one primitive tribe administered fierce red ants. From then until now, women have relied on folk remedies such as poisonous powders or soapy water, and "instruments" such as sticks and wire hangers. Early medical science developed ways to provoke miscarriage. None was very safe, most were painful, and all were traumatic.

Today, surgical abortion in the first three months of pregnancy can be safe, but it is still traumatic. In much of the world, if abortion is an option at all, the common method is dilation and curettage, D and C. The woman lies with her legs strapped into stirrups while a practitioner opens her cervix with a small rod. The opening is widened with a larger rod and then a still larger one. This dilation can take hours, often under anesthesia because of the pain. When the entrance is wide enough, the practitioner inserts a spoonlike device with a sharpened edge. With that, the fetus is scraped away.

Under sanitary conditions, with competent medical care, a D and C is quite safe. In many developing countries, or in illegal clinics in the back streets of cities where abortion is banned, the risk can be great. The uterus is easily perforated. Infection can set in and cause infertility. Every three minutes, a woman somewhere in the Third World dies from a badly performed abortion.

Altogether, well over 50 million abortions are performed each year, half of them illegally. The World Health Organization estimates that, as a consequence, 200,000 women die annually. In some countries, 50 percent of all maternal mortality is because of unsafe abortion. And for every woman who dies, another twenty to thirty suffer infections, uterine perforations, and lasting injuries often leading to sterility. The emotional toll is impossible to measure.

Where abortion is banned, practitioners find more primitive ways. Some thrust a stick into the womb until the fetus aborts, causing a torrent of bleeding. Others try violent abdominal massage. Often their purpose is to begin an abortion so that doctors, faced with the circumstances, will have to complete it.

The preferred modern method is suction. If performed within the first few weeks, under adequate conditions, it is a simple enough process. An instrument like a slender silver straw is slipped past the cervix without dilation. The doctor gingerly locates the fetus and then vacuums it away from the uterine wall.

In theory, a woman can drop into a clinic at eight o'clock and, after an hour's rest following the procedure, go on her way without another thought to her pregnancy. But it doesn't always work like that. She may begin hemorrhaging because of tissue left behind, or she may suffer the sharp pain of a perforation. Infection may set in, causing later distress and, in extreme cases, infertility. Even when the medical process is flawless, few women can simply shrug off the procedure. Any instrumental abortion is an intrusion. Physically, it is an operation and may leave a scar. Psychologically, it is an invasion of the most intimate reaches of a woman's body.

Only someone who has felt an embryo take root inside her womb can know the soaring hope or the deep dread of impending childbirth. From the first month, there are waves of fatigue and flashes of sickness. An eager mother absorbs these happily in anticipation of the new life to come. A reluctant one is likely to feel her world is collapsing around her.

Politicians and preachers seize abortion as an issue, seeking to define the beginning of life and set restrictions on how a woman can respond to the process at work in her body. Their definitions can only be arbitrary or emotional. Doctors agree that pregnancy starts with implantation, but no one can say when this *function* of human life becomes *a* human life. After the primitive streak, there is steady, continuous development.

The idea that fertilization leads necessarily to a human being is not scientifically sound. Far too much can happen to a zygote before it nests securely in the womb. More than half the time, zygotes miscarry spontaneously as a natural protection against birth anomalies. In any case, we do not know at what stage a *person* begins to exist. We probably will never know.

Any abortion represents a failure—an attempt to reverse a condition, correct a mistake, erase a reality. But as the Australian reproductive specialist Roger Short put it, abortion is like poverty: no one likes it, but it will always be with us.

For me, the challenge was clear. Medicine's mission is to help people. Why should 200,000 women die each year for lack of a better way? If science can make it otherwise, why must a woman's decision to terminate an unwanted pregnancy be accompanied by pain and punishment?

As a scientist who had studied hormones for all of his career, I knew there should be a better way. Rather than disrupt a pregnancy with a sharpened spoon or a suction tube, why couldn't the natural process be reversed by altering the balance of the same hormone that caused it to begin?

The answer was RU-486.

RU-486 is an antihormone, a muscular little molecule that interferes with hormonal messages. Its rival is progesterone. We devised it in 1980, with chemists and pharmacologists from the Roussel-Uclaf laboratories in Romainville, France, and we had more than abortion in mind.

Steroid hormones are messenger molecules that regulate reproduction, metabolism, and the body's responses to stress. Antihormones counter hormonal activity. And that was the crux of my research: to find a compound that would neutralize progesterone in the reproductive cycle.

When RU-486 was discovered, I knew we had a breakthrough in fertility control. At the same time, we had found an antihormone that could block the activity of cortisone-related hormones, which chemically resemble progesterone, with far-reaching implications for the treatment of diseases.

The detailed mechanism is complex, but the principle is simple. Hormones are transmitters. If their activity is blocked, their message is lost. RU-486's action is like jamming a radio signal.

Hormones function only if they bind with corresponding molecules, or receptors. Once the receptors in the target cells are identified, antihormones can be made to bind to them in the place of hormones. Hormones continue to be secreted normally; they simply cannot find anywhere to deliver their biological impulses, and thus trigger no action. RU-486 binds to the progesterone receptor and blocks the work of the hormone.

Another analogy makes this clear. In order to initiate action in the body, a receptor must be unlocked. The hormone is the key, and it must fit into a uniquely fashioned "keyhole" in the receptor. RU-486 is a false key. It enters the keyhole instead of progesterone. The progesterone may circulate, but it does so without effect. When RU-486 is no longer needed, it withdraws, leaving no trace in the body.

Deprived of progesterone action, the gestation process cannot continue. RU-486 breaks down the embryo's bond to the uterine wall. Without progesterone to calm the uterine muscle, contractions begin, and the cervix softens and widens. Menstrual-like blood flows, and the pea-sized embryo is washed from the body.

The expulsion is aided by another natural hormone in the uterus, prostaglandin. When a woman is given a small dose of synthetic prostaglandin after RU-486, the process is more than 95 percent effective up to five weeks after a missed period. If it fails, a woman can revert to a surgical alternative.

We are broadening RU-486's range in fertility control. The drug can also be taken in the second half of the menstrual cycle, before pregnancy begins. Blocking progesterone at that point triggers uterine bleeding so that a zygote cannot implant. Research continues toward using RU-486 as an oral contraceptive, preventing ovulation at midcycle.

Headline writers labeled RU-486 the "abortion pill." But there is no surgical invasion, no traumatic shock to the unwilling mother. In a sense, RU-486 is an unpregnancy pill.

More accurately, RU-486 is what I call a contragestive. Contraception prevents fertilization. Abortion excises a fetus. Contragestion works a middle range, countering gestation before implantation or in pregnancy's earliest stages. When used after implantation, RU-486 interrupts pregnancy. If taken earlier, it has the same effect as a morning-after pill.

To date, more than 80,000 women have used RU-486 in France. Britain and China have approved it, and other countries will follow. The procedure hardly amounts to a visit to a drugstore for a pill to pop, as some people first characterized it. In France, RU-486 is given only in approved family planning centers. But a woman's own doctor might just as easily guide her through the process, with expulsion occurring in her own home.

Recent research with prostaglandins is simplifying the procedure. When the technique was first introduced, women were required to return after forty-eight hours for an injection or a suppository, which could cause painful cramps. Even with the cramps, more than 80 percent of women who have experienced a surgical abortion as well as RU-486 say they prefer the pill. Further clinical trials have shown that women can take very small doses of a prostaglandin orally with the same efficacy and much less pain.

Eventually, a single pill containing both RU-486 and a time-release prostaglandin may reduce the drama of abortion to a simple, dignified encounter between a woman and her doctor. But even if the science is tidy, a woman's decision—however early—is not easily made.

Nearly a decade after its appearance, anti-abortion extremists still revile RU-486 as a "death pill." But each year, new research suggests more ways that the compound can protect life. Doctors use it in therapeutic abortions to spare mothers with deformed or diseased fetuses. In difficult deliveries, it can help avoid cesarean sections and give the newborn a better chance to survive.

Beyond the field of reproduction, it has proven effective in treating certain breast cancers, some inoperable brain tumors, and Cushing's syndrome. It is being studied for use against endometriosis, stress disorders, severe burns and wounds, and glaucoma. Future research may show RU-486 to have an impact on immunological disorders such as AIDS, and it may be helpful in alleviating some symptoms of menopause.

The oral contraceptive developed by Gregory Pincus was a revolution in the 1960s. This was, I believe, the first time that a medical discovery was perceived as changing human behavior. RU-486 is the next step. Its range of action falls between that of the pill, which altered women's lives decades ago, and conventional abortion, which is still their last resort. It is a contragestive, the second-generation pill.

I began as a doctor, and I remain a doctor, impassioned by a mission to heal. But a full-time bedside career would have left me no time to dream of discoveries and work toward bringing them to reality. From the start, I have been a doctor who practices science.

As the idea of RU-486 took shape, I felt a thrill not only as a doctor and a scientist but also as a man who believes an individual has a role in society. Here was a double chance: to help women preserve their health and shape their families and to help humanity on a wider scale, in addressing a demographic crisis that threatens to overwhelm us all.

Fertility control is at the heart of the human condition. Each of us must see it according to our values and sentiments. As for me, I have three children and seven grandchildren with an eighth on the way. I do not like abortion. But neither do I believe that women should be deprived of their most fundamental rights.

Margaret Sanger, who inspired Pincus to develop his pill, said it well: "No woman can call herself free who does not own and control her body." RU-486 can offer societies the means to safely limit their numbers by giving each woman control of her own body and the freedom to choose the size of her own family. And the poet Louis Aragon suggested why this is so important to us all: "Woman is the future of man."

Science imposes no solutions; it equips people with tools to fashion their own solutions. RU-486 is a means toward goals many of us share. It can change the way we look at fertility control. It can replace surgical abortion. Paradoxically, the "abortion pill" might even help eliminate abortion as an issue by the end of this century.

Chapter Two

THE
MORAL PROPERTY
OF WOMEN

RU-486 SLIPPED QUIETLY into the world, hardly stirring the higher echelons of France's scientific community. Then, suddenly, the pill and I were at the center of an international media storm. From the first presentation to the French Academy of Sciences, on April 19, 1982, RU-486 has clung precariously to a political roller coaster.

When the drug was ready for clinical trials, I chose the Cantonal Hospital in Geneva. Switzerland required that such tests be reviewed by an ethics committee. I was anxious for a reaction from a panel of citizens, beyond medical and scientific circles, to what was likely to be a political bombshell. At that time, France did not have such ethics committees.

I knew I could count on Walter Herrmann. During six years as head of gynecology and obstetrics at the University of Washington's hospital in Seattle, he spoke often and published widely. I was in close touch with him after he moved to chair the gynecology and obstetrics department at the University of Geneva, and always admired his calm and skillful manner. His tact and good sense were suited perfectly to the delicate job of testing RU-486.

Herrmann administered RU-486 to eleven women who were six to eight weeks pregnant. Nine aborted after four days. The drug failed in two cases, and the abortions were completed by routine aspiration. Normally a reserved man, Herrmann could not hide his excitement when he phoned me with his results.

The trials had determined that in terminating pregnancy, RU-486 could operate quickly and effectively. It showed other possibilities, too, but that much was proven. My colleagues and

I drafted an article for *Comptes Rendus,* the Academy's official journal, and I prepared to make the formal presentation. But there was a problem.

I had been elected to the Academy for my earlier work on steroid hormones, but was not yet registered as a member. Only members could publish in *Comptes Rendus.* As in the time of Louis XIV, the French head of state had to approve new academicians, and President François Mitterrand would not see the list before late spring.

Nonmembers had to transmit their articles through one of the chosen. I went to see Professor Jean Bernard, a leukemia specialist who is perhaps France's most revered scientist. He had nominated me to the Academy. Ascetic, often acerbic, Bernard had an imposing presence despite a slight stature and delicate, almost Oriental features. Then in his late seventies, he had been my mentor and friend for decades.

Bernard agreed to sponsor our findings and lend them the enormous weight of his name. But he saw the importance of our discovery, and thought it better that I introduce RU-486 myself so that I could answer questions. He proposed that to the Academy's governing council, and they agreed.

It was a daunting prospect. The Academy members were all specialists at the top of their fields. Few were biologists or physicians. The hall itself was forbidding—a magnificent chamber watched over by busts and portraits of the finest minds France had produced: philosophers, writers, artists, scientists.

The stuffy surroundings exuded tradition. The acoustics were terrible. A puny slide screen off to one side seemed out of place. I breathed deeply of the dust of three centuries, thought fleetingly of Lavoisier, Bonaparte, and Pasteur, and flung myself into the presentation. My audience was not visibly impressed.

I could only reveal part of the structure of RU-486 because the compound was protected by a commercial patent that would not be released for several more months. The diagram I presented had gray patches masking two appendages of the chemical formula. Although I produced a sealed envelope containing the missing information for the Academy's records, the secrecy of it all miffed some of my new confreres.

My report was noted with no trace of passion. From his raised podium, the permanent secretary of the Academy, Professor Robert Courrier, seemed in bad humor. Courrier was a complex man, with the robust, straightforward manner of a provincial farmer but a cunning sense for the politics of power within his field. He was a biologist who had spent years on his own hormone research.

Courrier passed over my main theme: the antiprogesterone effect on receptors and our breakthrough incorporating this into a new drug. "After all," he snorted, "this is abortion. Nothing more!"

His response reflected an uneasiness among members that avant-garde research had been applied directly to so delicate a human problem. Scientific breakthrough or not, abortion was in bad taste. I had not anticipated this problem, but I would face it again. It is almost impossible to speak of the science of reproduction without other considerations: political, moral, and ethical issues—everything from broad social concepts to petty prejudices.

This is understandable enough. Abortion stops life. To some, there is an inherent antithesis: abortion contradicts the reverence for life that we share as men and women as much as doctors. But that day I purposely stayed within the framework of explaining only my clinical results. It was not my place to expound on the rights of women or on questions of a metaphysical order.

Later, Bernard remarked only half in jest that it was lucky I had been elected a member before that day's presentation. It was a strange feeling. On the one hand I had been recognized by peers for my twenty-five years of hormone research. But I was also under fire. My scientific findings had stirred a bitter political controversy.

That was only the beginning. A reporter for Agence France-Presse who had been following my work wrote a dispatch that topped the front page of *Libération*, France's lively morning paper. It began: "A new method of regulating the female cycle, which might mean a serious alternative to current methods of contraception and abortion, was presented Monday to the Academy of Sciences."

The same morning, *The New York Times* filled the first page of its "Science Times" section with an article by Richard Eder. "A new birth control pill which women could take for four days at the end of each monthly cycle, instead of for three weeks as at present, has been devised by a leading French biochemist," Eder wrote. "Although Dr. Baulieu's work has been closely held, word of it has begun to arouse interest among several leading specialists in the United States and elsewhere."

Soon afterward, Pierre Salinger, tipped off by a mutual friend, brought over an ABC television crew. Other television cameras followed. Françoise Giroud wrote a glowing editorial in Milan's *Corriere della Sera.* My office at Bicêtre Hospital, on the southern outskirts of Paris, took on the ambience of a campaign headquarters on election night as I was grilled on television newscasts and interviewed by newspaper reporters.

The Associated Press relayed my findings to newspapers all over the world. Like *The New York Times*, AP seized on the aspect of taking the pill only at the end of the cycle.

From then on, the future of RU-486 was shaped as much by its exposure in the media as by its medical possibilities. Without coverage, this new discovery might have slipped by as only an interesting sidelight of science. But reporters immediately understood the drug's significance. In their coverage, however, they had to simplify their explanations, and a few of them inadvertently distorted the facts, causing some public confusion, which still remains. On the whole, press reaction was positive.

Thoughtful journalists saw the potential. Claudine Escoffier-Lambiotte, in *Le Monde,* described an essential point: "The early interruption of pregnancy by RU-486 is less traumatizing than aspiration or curettage and less toxic than massive doses of prostaglandins or estrogens (the 'morning-after' pill)."

Some of the reports were skeptical. Others beamed enthusiasm. *Le Nouvel Observateur* wrote, "Humanity impatiently awaits this marvelous new pill. Or rather anti-pill, par excellence." It quoted Yvette Roudy, a former minister of women's affairs, who compared me with Louis Pasteur. A companion article in the magazine, headlined "Bravo, But . . . ," tempered the euphoria by noting the limits of RU-486.

The World Health Organization and other international agencies took note of the media stir. Inevitably, every manner of activist weighed in. This was an encouraging sign. A full-blown debate, in which medical findings were disseminated along with moral, religious, and political considerations, seemed the best way for RU-486 to escape being a simple laboratory finding with no practical use.

None of this debate was lost on the people who owned the pill. Roussel-Uclaf's full designation for the compound was RU-38486, the total number of molecules synthesized by the company chemists until 1980. A lot of those discoveries had shown promise, but the company had to evaluate each as a viable product. Medical application was only part of the picture.

Roussel-Uclaf was widely known for political prudence. The firm's directors did not relish controversy. Hoechst A.G. of Germany, which owned a controlling interest, was even more cautious. As a large multinational corporation, Hoechst balanced a number of considerations in protecting its profits.

My own connection to RU-486 is only scientific. I am a professor at the public University of Paris South and director of a research unit at INSERM (Institut National de la Santé et de la Recherche Médicale), which is similar to the National Institutes of Health in the United States. I am also a part-time consultant to Roussel-Uclaf, and my work under their auspices belongs exclusively to them.

My arrangement with Roussel-Uclaf serves both sides. I can use the company's laboratories and testing facilities. They benefit from my ideas and findings. I receive a small fixed monthly retainer, with no royalties. If Roussel-Uclaf makes money from a product, I don't. If nothing comes of an idea which costs money to test, I lose nothing. This leaves me free to do independent research and, to speak my mind, as well as to exercise influence on an important pharmaceutical concern.

Edouard Sakiz, president of Roussel-Uclaf, was walking a

thin line. He had risen to the top as a leader who commanded respect and a biologist who knew his business. Staying there, however, took all of the skills of a consummate corporate manager. A former hormonal researcher, he was thrilled at the idea of RU-486. He also knew it was a very hot potato.

Sakiz never forgot a friend or broke with an enemy. He was crisply efficient, enamored of electronic wizardry. No papers cluttered his ornate art museum of an office. If facts were not memorized or computerized, they were forgotten. I first met him in the late 1950s, when he was a doctoral candidate from Turkey, a disciple of Courrier's. Courrier clashed with Roger Guillemin, who was then working in Paris and later won a Nobel Prize for medicine. Guillemin moved to Houston, and Sakiz followed. Later, Sakiz came back to France to work at Roussel-Uclaf.

Roussel-Uclaf's other directors were a complex mix of scientists and businessmen with differing philosophies. Before my presentation, they had discussed plans to test, license, and market the new product. After the flurry, this was no longer a corporate issue. All of them knew the world would be watching them closely.

There was some inevitable public confusion about RU-486, partly because I had not been clear enough and partly because reporters on deadline had to interpret a scientific paper for themselves. A few bestowed upon RU-486 a "morning-after" power: a quick fix, something a woman might take after lovemaking. Others hailed the end to a woman's need to saturate herself with hormones to ward off ovulation. Neither was quite right.

Testing showed that RU-486 taken near the end of the cycle could trigger menstruation, washing away a fertilized egg before it implanted firmly in the uterus. A woman who suspected imminent pregnancy could interrupt the process. In a broader sense, one might call that a "morning-after" capability.

But it is not so simple. Although RU-486 taken near the end of a fertile cycle is 80 percent effective in preventing pregnancy, the catch is that, in practice, it is reliable in this case only when used occasionally. RU-486 can affect the timing of the next cycle, lowering the chance of success in the following month. Even among women who are regular, vagaries in the menstrual cycle confound any systematic monthly hormonal method. Further research suggests promise that RU-486 eventually might be taken in ways that overcome this obstacle.

As stated earlier, this new method of menstrual regulation, neither contraceptive nor abortive, is contragestive. It does not stop fertilization, but it can act before pregnancy, which begins only when the blastocyst attaches itself and begins to develop in the womb. Or just after.

If the word *contragestion* is a mouthful for many people, it defines a little-understood range of birth control. This is shown in the accompanying diagram. Several existing methods, widely used but not well understood in how they actually work, correspond to the concept of contragestion. The intrauterine device, for example, is a double contragestive; it may prevent sperm from fertilizing the egg and a fertilized egg from implanting. Potentially, RU-486 could chemically replace all these methods.

Menstrual regulation or menstrual extraction refers to bringing on a late period with vacuum aspiration. This is done after the zygote implants, but it can be termed contragestion. Doctors prefer to wait up to eight weeks after a woman's last menses (when she is four weeks late) to do this procedure; before then, the embryo is difficult to locate. With RU-486, the process is more efficient: menstrual regulation can be done at any time through the ninth week, whether or not a pregnancy is confirmed.

To me, using RU-486 to dislodge an implanted embryo in its first weeks is also contragestion. But semantics are a separate issue. In the clinical results presented in *Comptes Rendus* we defined the method as abortion by medical means, without the use of instruments.

"Abortion" is a harsh term for a pill that eliminates the trauma of surgery. The word focuses on only a single dimension of RU-486's action. Still, "abortion" broke down all barriers of indifference. People reacted to the word. Our noisiest detractors helped us; in waving their flags they ensured that people would want to learn more.

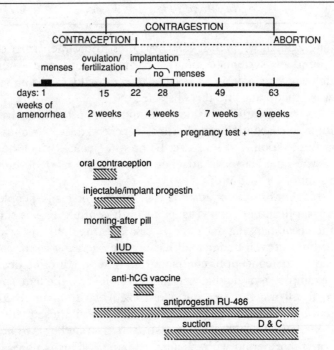

Contraception, Contragestion, and Abortion Birth control techniques range in time from methods preventing fertilization to the interruption of pregnancy at various stages. This chart shows the overlapping categories of several methods—classified as contraception, contragestion, and abortion—and their periods of efficacy, measured from the last menses.

Common terms are ambiguous. *Contraception* is usually understood to mean preventing fertilization, but specialists also refer to it until implantation is complete. To many biologists and theologians, *abortion* might mean any maneuver after fertilization; to practitioners, it is only after implantation. Most techniques can work in several ways. Even some oral contraceptives do not always block ovulation, for example; they can alter the endometrium and may prevent implantation, which is a post-ovulatory effect.

The diagram also shows *contragestion* from day 15, when fertilization takes place, to day 63, the limit until which RU-486 has been used for a voluntary interruption of pregnancy. It spans the time of other post-ovulatory methods.

Techniques are shown in shaded bars. Solid lines indicate the time when a method is most efficient. Dotted lines show when the method might also have some effect.

The American press made little distinction between contraception and abortion, let alone contragestion. All were lumped together as birth control. But the American reaction was enthusiastic, and specialists rallied around our discovery. Early supporters included Sheldon Segal, director of the population program at the Rockefeller Foundation and former head of the Population Council in New York.

Segal is one of those warmhearted, clear-thinking men who can inspire a movement. As a politician, he is a tireless advocate for new contraceptive methods, at the heart of an action network spanning the world. As a biologist, he is a driven researcher who spends his vacations poking into the reproductive habits of small animals.

At the time, he was preoccupied with Gossypol, a Chinese drug under study as a male contraceptive, and with Norplant, a female hormone implant which was approved for use in the United States in 1990. But he threw himself at RU-486. He set up a conference in Bellagio, Italy, in a lovely villa the Rockefeller Foundation lent to scholars, and we later edited a book together on the conference.

Officials at the World Health Organization also showed a strong interest, some of them spurred on by media attention. Alex Kessler, a friend for fifteen years, championed RU-486 within the U.N. agency. Kessler was a man of action, a charming and relaxed American with a huge capacity for work. He did not like to compromise.

Kessler directed WHO's Special Program of Research, Development, and Research Training in Human Reproduction, set up in 1972 to coordinate and evaluate research in the field. It was funded separately, with aid from Scandinavian countries, Canada, the World Bank, and other donors. He wanted to establish a network of international tests for RU-486, and I knew he could cut through WHO's bureaucratic maze.

At Roussel-Uclaf, Edouard Sakiz was overjoyed at WHO's interest. It was clear that RU-486 would have to be tested on a wide scale to gain credibility. Outside specialists had to observe and evaluate it. Sakiz doubted that he could persuade the company to find funds for such expensive and controversial trials. WHO would not only endorse the pill but also pay for its testing.

Kessler was just as delighted to find a product to test. He had been looking for an original, groundbreaking project since the inception of his program. His team of committed scientists had a specific mission. They wanted badly to make an important contribution in their field.

In 1982, Roussel-Uclaf signed an agreement with WHO to allow doctors to evaluate the drug under various conditions, in both developed and developing countries. If Third World public health services wanted to use it in clinics later on, the company would offer a reduced price. This would not only provide further research but also pave the way for RU-486's introduction into poorer countries.

One clause in the contract surprised me. It covered the eventuality that Roussel-Uclaf might decide not to develop the product even if a member nation of WHO wanted to use it. The company agreed either to provide RU-486 directly to the international organization or to cede rights to another manufacturer.

I asked Sakiz about this; he had been a friend and close colleague for years. Why would the company ever think of abandoning such an asset? "You never know," he replied. It took me some time to understand what was behind his enigmatic smile.

In the United States, Roussel-Uclaf reached an agreement with the Population Council, a nonprofit research organization with support from the Ford and Rockefeller foundations, among others. The accord gave the council rights to import RU-486 into the United States for large-scale testing. If RU-486 were approved by the Food and Drug Administration, the accord would make it possible for the drug to be distributed by a public, nonprofit organization such as Planned Parenthood.

C. Wayne Bardin, medical director of the Population Council, was intrigued. He obtained clearance from the Food and Drug Administration for abortion trials at the University of Southern California in Los Angeles.

In the meantime, Roussel-Uclaf worked on a basic strategy to bring the new discovery to the public. Any new drug can take five to ten years to develop in France, and decisions had to be made. If the WHO trials were successful, the company had a range of options. Sakiz wanted to market RU-486 aggressively. Others were reluctant, for both commercial and personal reasons. Some of them opposed abortion; a few wanted to depose Sakiz. Whatever their point of view, the directors knew that by now the pill had created too much of a stir to lie quietly in a drawer.

For the most part, the announcement of RU-486 caught scientific and medical circles by surprise. Researchers seldom keep up with each other's work except through specialized periodicals, with a lapse of time between submission and publication, or through infrequent professional conferences. This time, the news came by television and the morning paper.

My colleagues in France would have been peeved had they not received a full account in *Comptes Rendus*, available soon after my presentation to the Academy. Journals are a time-honored format. When a researcher leaks his findings before they are accepted in a scientific publication, others trot out the half-ironic, half-irritated observation: "He publishes in *Le Figaro*."

In the case of RU-486, my colleagues were forgiving. Intelligent men and women, they realized that something in a newspaper might, after all, be true or even important. Some doctors were instantly convinced. Misunderstanding the newspaper accounts, which confused initial tests with ready availability, they called for immediate supplies; women were demanding to be given RU-486.

In French hospitals, there were two reactions. One, simple and predictable, was positive. It came from clinical researchers in endocrinology who wanted to study the product scientifically as soon as possible to gain some distance on potential foreign competitors. The other reaction was negative. No major department of obstetrics and gynecology asked to experiment with RU-486 for abortion. The only volunteers for tests came from the Family Planning Association, which did not have a medical network, and from Dr. David Elia of the French students' health benefits association. Elia was the first French doctor to use RU-486.

The official response was mixed. Jacques Dangoumeau, director of pharmaceutical products in the Ministry of Health, was a little perturbed to learn about RU-486 in the newspapers. But he realized this was an experimental drug, not yet in his purview as a salable commodity. Its marketing could not be considered before results were confirmed and the regulatory process followed.

At Roussel-Uclaf, discord continued. Some executives lost no time calculating profits suggested by the sadly mounting number of surgical abortions. Several who had opposed a contraceptive pill fifteen years earlier, and who were dubious of profits from steroid research, suddenly changed their minds. Dedicated to the company, they were cheered by the commercial prospects and the free publicity. Other directors were critical, even hostile, because they opposed abortion. But in the beginning, despite the conflict, no one openly stood in the way.

A few Roussel-Uclaf researchers, with some reason, felt that the media did not pay enough attention to their role. I always took care to mention the principal collaborators in the drug's development. They all had signed the *Comptes Rendus* article. Unfortunately, journalists must simplify and shorten, and tend to focus on a single name known to the public. Reporters sought me out, and although I was a scientist who believed in teamwork, I took the opportunity to speak for RU-486. I quickly saw that media excitement would push our product forward.

The Roman Catholic Church, naturally enough, was not happy. Church officials condemned the pill, saying that while Catholicism favored scientific progress designed to relieve human suffering, it opposed contraception as well as abortion. It could only reject a product that had elements of both. They suggested that RU-486 would make abortion commonplace, more acceptable—or, as the French say it, "banalize" the termination of pregnancy.

This position was repeated by fundamentalists and extremists of right-to-life movements. To them, RU-486 only encouraged the sexual permissiveness they denounced with such vigor. This view has always troubled me. Abortion is a painful decision, never "banal." A pill cannot wipe out a woman's conscience. It is hardly what one critic depicted: a simple taking of "a few tablets left on the corner of the night table."

This argument, made so often by men, suggests to me a deep misunderstanding of women. Can one person impose his morality on another and force her to suffer the pain and mutilation of an outmoded scientific procedure? Can one human being deny another the right of choice? There is a certain conception of humanity in the balance here. Not to mention the medical tragedies of the Third World, which the Church deplores so vociferously.

It was obvious that we would face these questions eventually, but for the moment we had more specific challenges. RU-486, in the spring of 1982, was only a promising development with a successful clinical test. Our immediate concern was to make it into a drug available to doctors and their patients.

The next step was systematic analysis of the action of the compound in different applications. At Bicêtre Hospital, we examined the effects at varying phases of the female cycle, even after menopause. My old friend and associate, Paul Robel, helped direct research, along with Gilbert Schaison, an endocrinologist. Researchers in twenty countries used RU-486 in physiological studies of progesterone and corticosteroids. In the United States, federal law prohibited doctors at the National Institutes of Health from examining RU-486 as an abortion agent, but Lynn Loriaux, Lynnette Nieman, and their colleagues at NIH studied it as a possible contraceptive and as a treatment for adrenal disease.

Each species has its particular reproductive physiology, but the main hormonal processes are the same in all mammals. To understand what happens in humans, scientists study rodents and primates. Gary Hodgen, who directed maternity research for fifteen years at NIH, left in 1984 when Reagan administration policy not only deprived him of RU-486 but also foreclosed other valuable research. At new labs in Norfolk, Virginia, funded by the Jones Foundation, Gary's work with monkeys was decisive in helping to develop RU-486.

In 1984, WHO published the first results on RU-486 abortions in Sweden and Hungary. They confirmed Herrmann's findings: the compound was 80 percent effective in 42-day pregnancies. Our new challenge was to find a way to better the percentage.

At Roussel-Uclaf, we debated different dosages and ways of administering them. Injections were out because the compound is not easily dissolved. We knew that single doses were most convenient and simplest to supervise. André Ulmann, who organized the tests at Roussel-Uclaf, settled on 600 mg to be taken once orally, the dose still in use today. But the effectiveness rate remained around 80 percent. We needed a second compound to hasten and increase contractions. The obvious one was prostaglandin.

Sweden was the place to go. Sune Bergström and Bengt Samuelsson had won a Nobel Prize for pioneering the study of prostaglandins. With WHO help, their colleague Marc Bygdeman had studied abortions brought on by prostaglandins at Karolinska Hospital in Stockholm. Bygdeman is a cool, deliberate scientist with a Swedish bent for detail. He had examined prostaglandins' effects on muscle fibers in the uterus and on the dilation of the cervix.

Used alone, prostaglandins can induce an abortion. They are now used in the second trimester of pregnancy when a mother's health is at risk. But relatively high doses are necessary and cause painful contractions. The idea was logical: a measured use of prostaglandins should reinforce the action of RU-486. A light dose should work effectively and cause no complications, with little pain.

We were not alone in this idea. While Roussel-Uclaf was developing RU-486, Schering A.G. in Berlin was hard at work on a similar compound, also meant as an antiprogestin. Neither company was aware of the other's work at the time, but Roussel was first with the patent. The Schering people were unhappy at being beaten, but they developed a subtle strategy to look for other ways to move ahead. One was to use an antiprogesterone with prostaglandin.

When Roussel-Uclaf patented its new product, it did not

protect itself on this second step. There was a loophole, which Schering intended to exploit. But, as luck would have it, I was in Sweden for a conference in 1983 and praised the process—a joint Franco-Swedish achievement—in an interview with the Swedish newspaper *Dagens Nyheter* before I was aware of the German project. This brought the combined use of two compounds into the public domain, and Schering was not able to obtain exclusive rights to it.

Bygdeman organized trials on sixteen women. When I arrived for the Bellagio conference in October 1984, he pulled me aside. His sly smile, so out of character, revealed his triumph before he could tell me about it. By using RU-486 with a dose of prostaglandin that was five times less than that given alone to induce abortion, he had brought the success rate to 95 percent.

Later, David Baird, professor of reproductive endocrinology at the University of Edinburgh, conducted tests that confirmed the Stockholm results. Eventually, his trials among one thousand women in Britain proved RU-486 combined with prostaglandin to be effective up to sixty-three days after the last period. Our French group published the results in *Comptes Rendus* and the *New England Journal of Medicine,* and clinical confirmations poured in: from China, Holland, Spain, Italy, Finland, the United States, Hungary, Singapore.

André Ulmann and Catherine Dubois at Roussel-Uclaf began drafting a dossier in French and English to be submitted in any country to apply for a distribution license. A French version, with the necessary documents to seek approval for administering RU-486 alone at 600 mg, was ready by the summer of 1987.

At the time we had little idea of how deeply anti-abortion activists feared our work. Dr. John Willke, then president of the National Right to Life Committee in the United States, established an international federation with headquarters in Lausanne and an office in Rome. In June 1987, in a letter to Prime Minister Jacques Chirac, he described alleged dangers of RU-486 and its "fetotoxicity." After a second letter in December, the Ministry of Health replied that all evidence would be weighed when a decision was taken on a license for the product.

Willke denounced RU-486 as "chemical warfare on the unborn." This distorted the facts, since the compound has no effect on the fetus itself. It acts physically to separate the fetus from the uterine wall. With less trauma to the mother, it does what any surgical abortion does.

Most of the heat was generated outside of France. French *"Laissez-les vivre"* (Let them live) committees held news conferences and issued protests, but their impact was so slight that I did not hear about them until later. We were too busy at the time finishing our official dossier. On October 9, 1987, Laboratoires Roussel, a division of Roussel-Uclaf, applied for a license to market "mifepristone," the generic name for RU-486; the company's French brand name was Mifegyne.

The application was for RU-486 *alone*, without prostaglandin, and its stated purpose was to terminate pregnancy within two weeks after a missed period. Women could now have a medical alternative to suction or D and C. Conforming to the 1975 French abortion legislation, known as the Veil law, it specified an effectiveness of 80 percent. In case of failure, women could fall back on surgical methods.

The French law, proposed by Health Minister Simone Veil, allows women to opt for an abortion through the tenth week after a missed period. It is not a matter of securing permission from doctors, and indeed a doctor who refuses on the grounds of conscience must refer her to someone else. Under a compromise among legislators, a woman must observe a seven-day "period of reflection" between the time she announces her intention and her abortion. Additionally, the abortion must take place at one of France's 850 authorized family planning centers.

The law's strength is that it requires a woman to make her decision early, before she is ten weeks late, which is twelve weeks after fertilization. This is when progesterone starts being secreted by the placenta, no longer by the ovaries. This date does not mark any distinct change in the continuum, but the twelve-week limit has a certain scientific and philosophical sense since the product of conception by now has acquired more hormonal independence.

We expected the ministry's commission of specialists to approve the dossier within three months. In the meantime, we continued with tests in France and Britain to add a small dose of prostaglandin to improve the effectiveness, hasten expulsion, and reduce bleeding.

A month after our application, the National Ethics Committee for Health and Life Sciences began preparing for its annual December meeting. RU-486 would be on the agenda. Jean Bernard was head of the consultative committee, and so I was optimistic. Bernard had known me since I was a resident. I often sat next to him at Academy meetings to savor his witty, sage, and often severe asides. I told him about the recent successes in prostaglandin tests, and he suggested I hurry the data into *Comptes Rendus* to get it on the record.

The Ethics Committee bans the public from its deliberations but issues communiqués and briefs the press on its opinions. Its decisions are not binding on officials. But as it is composed of a weighty blend of scientists, jurists, religious and civic leaders, and government representatives, its advice is seldom ignored. Noting the 95 percent success rate with prostaglandin in British and French trials, the committee pronounced itself in favor of RU-486. Not unanimously, however. Some members objected, saying that the method enabled women to act too quickly, to make a decision on pregnancy they might later regret.

Although I was happy with the result, the newspapers seized on the resistance. "Yellow light for RU-486," reported *Le Parisien*. "Yes But . . . for RU-486," said *Le Figaro*. In fact, the Ethics Committee's only hesitation was their stipulation that the pill be used in approved centers rather than being sold in drugstores or supermarkets. This seemed very appropriate to me. Although taking a pill requires far less supervision than surgery, anything relating to pregnancy must be controlled. It is only natural to continue to respect the law on abortion when using a drug instead of an instrument.

Though the media frenzy was mostly positive, it worried me. I was afraid the Ministry of Health commission members might be irked by so much publicity, taking it as pressure on them. By coincidence, their deadline for a decision was only weeks after the Ethics Committee meeting. And they were looking at an outmoded dossier, one that did not include results on prostaglandin. The situation was delicate. Even with the Ethics Committee's decisive vote, a single negative opinion could sway the balance at the ministry.

The commission met on January 15, 1988, and remarked favorably on the dossier. But rather than accept published reports from the Academy of Sciences and the authoritative British medical journal *Lancet,* where Baird had published, the commission demanded more information on the use of prostaglandin. *France-Soir* phrased it, "Morning-After Pill Put Off to After the Morning-After."

Such delays were standard procedure; they did not necessarily suggest medical or administrative resistance. But RU-486 was getting to be a notorious molecule. Unavoidably, some sectors interpreted the delay as political, and the heat was turned up on both sides. The French presidential elections were approaching in March. Perhaps strategists for Jacques Chirac, who opposed Mitterrand, felt that this was no time to endorse such a controversial product.

We were getting used to this trepidation by now. We knew it would not be long before the first enthusiastic headlines gave way to the inevitable, like a later one in the *Times* of London which read: "A Bitter Pill to Swallow."

Roussel-Uclaf produced a new dossier in mid-March 1988, but the commission was not ready to study it before May. Since France is largely paralyzed in the summer months, the commission decided to meet on RU-486 in September.

During the delay, opposition forces gathered their strength. Roussel-Uclaf stockholders' meetings were not noted for liveliness, but the June 23 assembly seethed revolution. Scores of protesters besieged the sedate corporate headquarters on the Boulevard des Invalides. Some were dressed as World War II deportees, evoking the poison gas manufactured for Adolf Hitler by Hoechst's predecessor company, I.G. Farben. They shouted slogans as directors walked past: "Assassins, stop your work of death!" And "You are turning the uterus into a crematory oven!" Tracts described RU-486 as a chemical weapon destined to "poison the still-tiny children of a billion Third World mothers." Inside, the audience included Dr. Xavier Dor of Pitie-Salpetrière Hospital, a crusader against abortion. Borrowing an American tactic for disrupting shareholders' meetings, he bought a single share of Roussel-Uclaf stock as an entry ticket.

The demonstrators did not worry me. Clinical trials of RU-486 and prostaglandin were fast expanding, showing successful results in far more cases than necessary for application. Roussel-Uclaf offered the compound free to researchers around the world, and their body of data was overwhelming. Confirming my optimism, someone sent me a copy of the natural sciences final examination at the staid Versailles Academy. In one of the exam questions, students at the level of high school seniors were asked about RU-486, extraordinary for such a new discovery. Confident of success, I devoted my attention to other work at my research laboratory, INSERM.

At Roussel-Uclaf, however, hands were wringing. A campaign in the United States deluged the French Embassy in Washington with letters threatening boycotts against French products. They demanded official action to stop the development of RU-486. Ambassador Emmanuel de Margerie himself was not alerted. Instead, an aide who screened the embassy's mail simply sent a memorandum to the Foreign Ministry. A ministry official, apparently with dubious intentions, relayed the note personally to Christian d'Aumale, a former ambassador who had been named by the state as chairman of the board of Roussel-Uclaf.

The state's role in the company was delicate. When the Socialist government targeted ten large companies for nationalization, Roussel-Uclaf was on the list. Hoechst, the main shareholder, said it would raise no objections, but in that case, it would separate the French company from its lucrative multinational structure. As a compromise, the French government acquired only a 36 percent equity interest in Roussel and the right to name a chairman.

D'Aumale had no direct power to derail the application.

Still, he had a certain influence. And he spread alarm among the other directors, who were already a little nervous from the stockholders' meeting.

At the time, I was off to Japan to talk about RU-486 at a scientific meeting. Not thinking about distances, I agreed to stop off first in Chile to speak at an international culture conference opposed to President Augusto Pinochet's heavy hand. When I finally dragged myself into Kyoto, André Ulmann reached me by telephone. "They're stopping everything," he said, his voice breaking with emotion.

The company directors had decided to withdraw their application for a license. They would cancel the development of RU-486 and halt distribution to centers that had continued to use it after the first trials. Ulmann asked me to appeal to Sakiz. I immediately called the president's assistant and confidante, Catherine Euvrard. She was a gifted neurobiologist who, like Sakiz, was a partisan of the pill.

Hoarsely, I pleaded my case. How could we deprive women of a drug that would spare them pain and potential danger? How could Roussel abandon RU-486 when such a discovery comes along at most once a decade? How could we demoralize our researchers like this? How could Sakiz be trapped by ambitious directors who wanted him to fall?

Sure there were risks in proposing a compound that had such social and moral implications, but how could directors, after investing so much money and expressing such great hope, suddenly decide to abandon it? Without medical justification, the impression would be that RU-486 had been somehow defective.

A free-for-all followed in late July. Finally, the divided managers and directors consulted Pierre Joly, number two in the company, who was vacationing in Corsica. Affable and intelligent, a pharmacist, Joly was respected by international peers for his ethical business sense. There was no going back, he said. The company might demur for commercial reasons when it came time to market the product. But RU-486 would have to await official validation. Withdrawing an application was inconsequential, he remarked.

The group's third-ranking officer, a mathematician named Alain Madec, wanted to drop RU-486 entirely. He was a former adviser to the Ministry of Industry and was educated at the classic fount of ranking French civil servants, the Ecole Nationale d'Administration. Madec was thought to reflect government thinking. Colleagues suspected him of personal ambitions, seeking to unseat Sakiz as president.

It was August, and Paris took on its summer air of a ghost town. The streets were empty except for tourists and Frenchmen who had put their troubles on hold. I was in a state of high anxiety, about to leave on holiday as the fate of our discovery hung by a thread. When I called Sakiz for news, he suggested lunch.

Catherine Euvrard, Sakiz, and I sat down to a fine meal. The application would stand, they announced. We finished some excellent wine, and I went to the airport reassured. The future of RU-486 was safe. If granted a license for sale in France, I was sure it would find its own way against all other obstacles.

On September 23, 1988, a Friday, RU-486 was officially approved for distribution in France. This time, *France-Soir*'s headline was: "The Morning-After Pill Is for Today."

It was a good week. On Monday, I'd been told that Chinese authorities also approved it. The product would be used not only in my own country but also in a nation that constituted nearly one quarter of humanity. I kept the Chinese decision to myself, fearing that huge headlines, only days before the French ministry had to pass judgment, would only seem like more pressure.

Later that week, I was in Bethesda, Maryland, addressing a conference at NIH, but my speech, intended to be rich in nuance and complexity, was delivered through clenched teeth. Emotion kept creeping into my sober scientific presentation. Newspaper and radio reporters called me, one after another, on a telephone beside the podium. Antenne 2, a major French network, brought in cameras.

I was worried that this could create a diplomatic incident, because the network was owned by the state, and the Reagan administration was dead set against abortion. RU-486 abortion research was banned at federal facilities, including NIH. But it seemed no one in America saw fit to try to censor a discussion of science.

We were pleased with the media interest, but even more warming were the reactions of Solomon Sobel, director of metabolism and endocrine drug products at the Center for Drug Evaluation and Research at the Food and Drug Administration, and his associate, Philip Corfman. They asked for a dossier on RU-486 so they could be prepared when an application was made in the United States.

Others were not so pleased. On an ABC television program, I found myself opposite a right-to-life activist whose remarks were closer to insults. I shrugged off most, but one left me stupefied: "You are a very good scientist," he said. "We will gladly give you money for research if you will help stop all spontaneous miscarriages." This is an instance of nature correcting its own mistake, expelling a defective fetus. Probably more than half of all fertilized eggs are eliminated in this way. It is nature's way of protecting the species. My interlocutor wanted to reverse that process to comply with his own reading of the will of God.

Polemics flew in France, naturally enough. But there were more ominous rumblings in Germany. Hoechst, which owns 54 percent of Roussel-Uclaf, was extremely hostile. Wolfgang Hilger, the president of Hoechst, came to Paris in October for a concert directed by Herbert von Karajan to celebrate the twentieth anniversary of Hoechst's association with Roussel. Hilger, a devout Catholic, reviled abortion. He would not talk to me and, later, refused to see me in Frankfurt.

I went back to work in my lab, a little busier than usual in light of events. The essential part—the application—was done; we had only to take the necessary steps to put RU-486 on the market. At the time, my overriding concern was Roussel-Uclaf's participation at the World Congress of Gynecology and Obstetrics in Rio de Janeiro, two years in the planning.

Every three years, specialists meet under the aegis of the International Federation of Gynecology and Obstetrics (FIGO).

That year, 9,500 people would attend. As other major pharmaceutical companies often do, Roussel-Uclaf sponsored a session. It was planned for October 27, and the theme was antiprogesterone. I would preside, aided by Sheldon Segal, with presentations by Marc Bygdeman and David Baird, Dr. Vera Hingorani of New Delhi, Dr. Zheng Shu-Rong of Beijing, and others. It was RU-486's moment.

In France, the situation was bubbling. The Catholic Church spoke out against the licensing of RU-486. Angry letters poured into Roussel headquarters. The general climate in Paris did not bode well. Catholic extremists protested Martin Scorsese's film *The Last Temptation of Christ*. They set a fire in the St. Michel Cinema, which injured thirteen people.

I was preoccupied, hurrying to prepare for Rio and finish other work. On the day of my departure, I finally reached Catherine Euvrard, who had been trying to call me for days. She said, in her habitual cheerful tone, that Sakiz wanted to see me but did not say why. I was busy, I said, and could make time only at the end of the day on my way to the airport. That was fine, she said, but her note of urgency troubled me. Later, I was told that Sakiz had tried to call me. Something was up. That afternoon, I found out what it was.

An assistant walked into my lab, ashen, and handed me a communiqué. It read:

"In the face of emotion on the part of public opinion in France and abroad and in the face of a polemic incited by the possibility of using the [drug for] abortions, Roussel-Uclaf has decided to suspend, starting today, the distribution of this product as a medical alternative to surgical abortion in France and abroad."

The announcement would be made public as soon as Sakiz knew that I had seen it. Ironically, after all the efforts made to obtain the registration of the compound, the company was giving up.

On the Friday before the Rio congress, Roussel-Uclaf's directors had discussed RU-486. Some spoke passionately in defense of the product; others damned it as an invitation to trouble.

Behind it all was a crisis with Hoechst, which wanted nothing to do with the immoral molecule.

Opponents warned of possible boycotts of Roussel-Uclaf products, extending perhaps even to Hoechst's wares. RU-486 was not worth the risk. The drug did not promise enormous profits. It would be ordered mainly by governments in developing countries and, therefore, sold at low prices fixed by WHO. Roussel was wasting its time with a product that threatened its internal peace, they argued. Some employees, after all, opposed abortion.

Defenders countered that Roussel-Uclaf should not give in to blackmail from a minority. The disputed compound conformed exactly to the therapeutic principles of the company; retracting it would obstruct the development of related products, and that would be a loss to medical science. The company had a social obligation to fulfill. What about all the researchers and technicians who had worked so hard to develop the molecule? What would they think of a cowardly last-minute about-face?

Euvrard, the only woman present among nineteen men, spoke out courageously on behalf of a product she had watched take shape. In this matter, she said, the company's attitude toward women was "indefensible."

After an hour, Sakiz called for a vote. He phrased it in negative terms. Are you for or against the suspension of RU-486? By a vote of sixteen to four, the "fors" carried it.

The assistant who brought me the news was amazed that I was not furious. I try hard to stay calm when faced with nasty surprises. While she fumed and stamped around for me, I looked for a way to fix this stupidity.

I studied the communiqué, which concluded: "Roussel-Uclaf is considered one of the pioneers in endocrinology. After having developed numerous hormones (sexual steroids and corticosteroids), it has oriented its research toward antihormones and their applications. Thus nilutamide (anti-androgen) has been recently placed at the disposal of the medical profession to treat patients suffering from prostate cancer. Roussel-Uclaf, convinced of the therapeutic value of antihormones, intends to continue its efforts in research and development in this field to maintain its scientific lead at a world level."

Between the prudently drafted lines, I could sense a bad conscience. Sakiz's motives had to be complex. He must have known he was standing against the current; RU-486 would stay its course, no matter what. He would have to face serious questions. In France, 150 centers were already using the pill and would fight to keep it. How would he explain the reversal to WHO? And how could researchers be motivated to continue their work, as the communiqué promised, if the company threw out their successes?

I found Sakiz in his office, visibly shaken. I can still see him: taut and pale, ill at ease in a somber suit. Suspending RU-486 was a matter of conscience, he said. The compound had brought nothing but trouble. Charged with emotion, he evoked his responsibility to the staff. He mentioned the fire at the St. Michel Cinema; he had to protect employees from a similar assault. My situation was different from his, he said, and I should react in any way I saw fit.

The decision affected women's rights and health, I said, and when the public learned of it the directors' prestige would suffer. Suspending RU-486 might destabilize the company rather than strengthen it. Future research would suffer. I predicted the derision that would soon follow: The satirical weekly *Le Canard Enchaîné* mocked the board and accused Alain Madec of angling for Sakiz's job.

Sakiz told me of strong disapproval from Hoechst-Roussel Pharmaceuticals Inc. (HRPI), the joint subsidiary in the United States, itself a branch of Hoechst Celanese Corporation, the American arm that brings in a quarter of Hoechst A.G.'s worldwide earnings. The companies, convinced that marketing RU-486 would tarnish their image, wanted no part of it. That had weighed heavily on Sakiz's decision.

After fifteen minutes, we had no more to say. Our old mutual esteem tempered any bitterness, and he wished me bon voyage. He asked if it wasn't a little crazy to go so far for two days. Had Sakiz forgotten that I was going to Rio to promote

RU-486? Or did he foresee what was likely to happen while I was in Rio? He confided to me that he hoped the decision would provoke a strong reaction from French authorities or the general public. But, he added, he alone could do nothing.

I wondered if Sakiz was subtly encouraging me to tell the world how I felt. He knew I was an independent sort. Later, some people suspected that we had cooked up a clever maneuver to take the matter to the public, but that wasn't the case. We each played our part, and acted according to our own consciences. I defended RU-486 openly. He did it in his own way.

I arrived in Rio to introduce RU-486 at the same moment Roussel-Uclaf announced in France that it was off the shelves. Three company colleagues burst into my hotel room. They had been there for three days. Seething with anguish but obliged to keep silent, they had answered a barrage of technical questions as if nothing was wrong. André Ulmann was particularly sickened. He felt that some Roussel executives had played the Hoechst card to please the parent company; their careers would last longer than Sakiz's.

The news hit the meeting like a bomb. Journalists clamored for interviews. Before replying, I met with my colleagues. They found me too optimistic, not recognizing the gravity of the situation. I insisted that this was a minor setback. To my mind, RU-486 was impossible to stop.

I made the same points again and again. The decision contradicted the advice of the Ethics Committee and Ministry of Health officials who granted the license, I said. Yielding to intolerance was morally scandalous. No imperative can block the progress of medical science in contributing to the well-being of patients. The Catholic Church's reference to the "banalization" of abortion—that such a simplified technique would make abortion commonplace, or banal—was an insult to women.

An international chorus joined in protest. In New York, Faye Wattleton of the Planned Parenthood Federation of America gave the company directors a taste of what they might expect if they thought giving in to the anti-abortionists would avoid controversy. She called their decision "a tragic display of cowardice and a shocking blow to women around the world."

Sheldon Segal, among others, found it "inappropriate" to block the use of a new drug for other than medical reasons, touching off a chorus of seconding opinions from specialists all over the globe.

At the Hotel Nacional, the scene was surreal. Roussel-Uclaf's display took up the lobby, a temple to their sacrificed molecule. Physicians and reporters fought for space, yelling questions. Finally, we moved to the press room for an impromptu briefing. I batted down an ugly rumor: infants had not been born deformed because of RU-486.

In Brazil alone, there are more than four million illegal abortions a year. Tens of thousands of women die or are maimed for life by clandestine operations, and doctors today report that the crisis is getting worse. Brazilian colleagues were anxious to learn more about RU-486 in a country still awaiting legalized abortion, with a desperate shortage of medical and surgical staff.

I received a telex from a group of companies in Oman. They would put up the capital to build a plant in China to synthesize RU-486 so that it could be distributed around the world. Was RU-486 to become a Sino-Arab hybrid?

In light of events, our sideshow presentation grew into a general assembly. We moved it to the main hall, and four thousand people jammed inside. I asked speakers to deliver their prepared texts with no changes. I wanted facts, only facts, at a working session, though it was perhaps a little too scientific for all the journalists who came.

It was a passionate event. Bygdeman, Baird, and Zheng reported on new successes. Vera Hingorani spoke of the enthusiasm of Indian women. Two hours passed in a flash, and reporters demanded more. In personal reflections, researchers lamented Roussel-Uclaf's decision. Zheng said Chinese hospitals would have to return to more onerous, traumatizing methods.

Ideas were floated for distributing RU-486. A nonprofit organization might be set up to buy the patent; if it marketed nothing else, a boycott would have no effect. China might make the drug under license. The most promising course should have been WHO, which had rights under the 1982 protocol. But the WHO representative replied cautiously. Given its levels of bureaucracy, a United Nations agency was not a likely candidate.

Directors of FIGO, who had organized the conference, wrote a protest letter to Wolfgang Hilger at Hoechst. He replied that abortion was morally reprehensible. RU-486 did not fit with the philosophy of his company. Hilger neglected to mention the responsibility, also moral, of any pharmaceutical company: to furnish a product when doctors ask for it because they judge it to be beneficial.

FIGO's position was crucial, since the organization deals with all matters affecting reproduction. Generally, FIGO directors try to reconcile each new scientific advance with the daily work of practitioners. They had just published a study on maternal mortality, finding that more than 500,000 women died from pregnancy-related causes each year, 99 percent of them in the Third World. They sought to cut that toll in half by the year 2000. That modest goal suggested the difficulty of the task. RU-486 could help.

The Rio conference produced unanimous support for the pill, from renowned specialists to village doctors. An entire profession attuned to women expressed deep concern. The movement born that day not only rallied behind RU-486, with which few doctors had practical experience, but strongly censured the notion that a pharmaceutical company can abandon a drug for nonmedical reasons. Roussel's act had violated the doctor's right to prescribe a proven method, as well as the patient's right to choose it.

Most doctors agree that pharmaceutical companies should be in a position to make profits so that those companies can afford to develop new drugs. But if a company chooses not to market a helpful product, it should give up its rights. There is no justification for locking away a scientific breakthrough.

I was touched by the flood of support, so different from the more typical quiet processes of science. It was a reward for our work, but it was more. Here was evidence that scientific research is valued by large numbers of people, who pour out their appreciation if they see how it contributes to their lives. And I chuckled at the irony. Inadvertently, Roussel-Uclaf had mounted a gigantic publicity campaign for RU-486 and its creators. The international press, television networks, specialized publications, and humanitarian associations from around the world saw—whether one was for RU-486 or against it—a triumph of French scientists. The Roussel-Uclaf directors had sought to escape criticism. Instead, they were pilloried on the front page of *The New York Times*.

Worn out by the tumult, I roamed Rio's botanical gardens and marveled at insect-eating plants. The encounter of two living worlds, plant and animal, always moves me. At the zoo, I discovered a curious animal called a tamandua, a tropical anteater with a head the size of two walnuts, a long neck like a little giraffe, and bearlike paws that seemed at once brutal and tender. Nature's lack of logic amused the biologist in me. Soon enough, I'd again be facing an absence of logic in human affairs.

The next morning, packed for the flight home, I got a call from Brigitte Castelnau of Agence France-Presse. The situation in Paris was paralyzed, she said. No one knew what would happen next. Minutes later, the phone rang again. It was another AFP reporter. I told him I had just hung up with his agency and suggested testily that they might organize themselves better. He waited for my tirade to subside, then told me the news. Health Minister Claude Evin had just revived RU-486.

Evin's declaration had been blunt: "From the moment governmental approval for the drug was granted, RU-486 became the moral property of women, not just the property of a drug company." If Roussel-Uclaf did not market the product, rights would go to a company that would.

Before we left Rio, we opened the champagne.

I am not sure what happened in Paris to prompt Evin's action. The press played a part. So did women's groups. Former health minister Michèle Barzach declared herself shocked by the sus-

pension. Eminent doctors objected, including Léon Schwarzen-
berg, himself a former health minister. In any case, Evin was on
solid ground. The government owned a third of Roussel-Uclaf
stock, and so it had some say. More important, a 1968 law holds
that if a company refuses to make a drug available, the health
minister can withdraw its license and award it to another company.

Soon after Evin's statement, Roussel-Uclaf put Mifegyne
back on the market, and it remained there. The ministerial stand
was not an order. By law, Evin would have had to ask approval
of the Ministry of Industry and call a commission to review the
case. But his *coup de force* demonstrated the power of an idea
whose time has come. Roussel's Pierre Joly admitted a sense of
relief. "We have thrown off what for us had become a moral
burden," he remarked at one point. "It was not up to us to come
between those who are in favor of abortion and those who are
against."

Our next step was to win authorization abroad, even as we continued research into the drug which had caused such an uproar.
I had no commercial stake in the pill. It had been a joint effort,
developed over years in France and perfected in several countries. But my name was on it, and the banner was mine to carry.

As time went on, my office at Bicêtre Hospital accumulated
nearly a ton of documents, mail, and press clippings. One letter,
addressed to "Garbage," suggested that I roast in hell. But an
article in *Parents* magazine hailed a "second revolution" in birth
control, a successor to Gregory Pincus's contraceptive pill of the
1960s. That thought touched me deeply. I had come down a long
road, in the steps of a great man.

Chapter Three

THE
ROAD TO
RU-486

GREGORY GOODWIN ("GOODY") PINCUS strode distractedly through our somber, cavernous medical school building on the Rue des Saints-Pères, and I was not particularly impressed. It was 1957, and he had come to Paris for a conference. Pressed for time, he visited the medical faculty only briefly. We all crowded into the hall for a look. A colleague explained some things in feeble English, and Pincus merely nodded his great Einsteinian head. His thick, bushy eyebrows bunched in a frown. He was not tall, but he stood ramrod straight, hardly noticing anyone around him. After a few perfunctory handshakes, he was gone.

Four years later, it was all different. I had found a way to detect a particular hormonal substance secreted by the adrenal glands, dehydroepiandrosterone sulfate. This discovery had eluded Thadeus Reichstein, who isolated cortisone and most of its related hormones, and other great chemists. I did it with a simple idea which, in classical terms, made little sense.

When adrenal glands are cancerous, dehydroepiandrosterone (a fatty steroid) appears in large quantities as a sulfate in urine. The accepted thinking was that the elusive substance could be traced back through the oily fluids from the adrenal glands. That seemed reasonable. But until then, scientists had looked for it in vain by examining the fat-based content of extracts taken from the adrenals. I decided to try the water phase in search of the sulfate form, which is water-soluble. It was like probing a vinaigrette: looking in the vinegar instead of the oil.

This pursuit taught me as much about scientists as science.

It was a question of rank and order. To scientists, the adrenal glands are noble. Urine, containing waste products such as sulfates, is only interesting to clinical chemists, not to "real" biologists.

My discovery caught the attention of everyone in the field, especially those in reproduction control who follow progress in the steroid hormones that control sexual function. Gregory Pincus asked me to speak at his Worcester Foundation, near Boston, the Mecca of hormone specialists. And it was Pincus who changed my life. He headed me down the long road toward RU-486 without even realizing it.

I was spending a year in the United States. Seymour Lieberman, a giant among biochemists, had invited me to work with him at Columbia University. My dehydroepiandrosterone sulfate discovery had enabled him to recalculate a crucial series of experiments, advancing work that had gone off track. His laboratory was on the sixteenth floor of Presbyterian Hospital on 168th Street, in a neighborhood of poor eastern European and German immigrants. By the time I went to Worcester, I had learned a lot about the world beyond France. Simply getting to America, in my situation, was an adventure.

In France, the notion of a sabbatical year did not exist for young professors. Having tenure, I was able to break away but only after finding colleagues to teach my biochemistry classes. Then there was the question of a visa. As a youth in the French Resistance against the Nazis, I had joined the Communist party. Although I quit after the Russians crushed the Hungarian uprising in 1956, it took some convincing for American authorities to realize that I had no subversive activities in mind.

For two years, the Eisenhower administration refused my visa application. Lieberman and others appealed on my behalf. They explained that I could help fill in a piece to a vital puzzle. Immigration officials were not moved. Then John F. Kennedy was elected in November 1960. Within weeks of his inauguration, I was on board the *Liberté*, on its last voyage to New York.

Friends I met on the voyage introduced me to a different world. Barbara Rose, the art critic, took me in hand and put me in my place. On my first day in Manhattan, she walked me down

Fifth Avenue. I glanced at the windows and observed mildly that, yes, they were all right but Paris also had beautiful things. Barbara laughed and nailed me in her impeccable French: "Stop playing the petit français."

I stayed in Terry Brook's apartment off Central Park and noticed a small painting, a white labyrinth on a blue background signed by Frank Stella. I was introduced to Stella, little known at the time, and fell into the circle of Jasper Johns, Robert Rauschenberg, Andy Warhol, and other pioneers of pop art.

These young artists were not bothered by the lack of foie gras at their parties. They traveled little and worked all the time. None was as yet rich and famous. Acclaim would come later, from the steadily expanding flow of their talent. Looking back, I am pleased at early premonitions of my friends' success. I never collected their paintings, though certain of their eventual value. Instead, I wanted to keep the material side separate from my feeling for their creative spirits at work. That was what bound us together.

I realized from my artist friends the similarity of creation in science and art. Like them, I was adding form to a blank space with only vague notions of where it would lead me. They understood little of what I did, and they could not purchase the product of my work. But we recognized a common spirit, and we were all confident of heading somewhere important.

Finding Seymour Lieberman was a lesson in the particular humility of scientific stars. Viewed from France, he was a deity, and I had assumed that each morning he had to brush aside torrents of accolades. When I got to Presbyterian Hospital, no one knew him. Eventually, after being pointed here and there, I knocked on the door next to his laboratory and asked for the great doctor. "Who?" said the white-coated researcher inside.

Lieberman dominated the international field of steroid research and took every opportunity to promote the work of the young French *protégé* on his team. From him, I learned to rejoice in the triumph of my students, which is not always easy for a professor-researcher; feeding his ego is often a researcher's only reward.

He taught me never to publish successes in a form so brief

that only the positive results are covered. He also showed me the value of controls to guard against results marred by chance or technical errors. For Lieberman, it was a moral imperative of scientists to publish all of their findings, even when inconclusive, mediocre, or negative. What a scientist observes might help others, and therefore science, even if he derives no benefit.

More than a mentor, Lieberman, forty-five at the time, was both a big brother and the father I never got to know.

I was born in Strasbourg but hardly ever lived there. My father, named Léon Blum, like the French Socialist statesman, died before I was four. He was an Alsatian born in 1874 under German occupation. A physician specializing in kidney disorders, he had also studied chemistry and earned a doctorate in science at Berlin. He was drafted into the German army in 1914 and was awarded an Iron Cross. But, like most Alsatians, he was passionately French. His medical activities allowed him to even the balance. Under the pretext of following cases, he asked officers he treated to send frequent postcards detailing the quantity of their urine. From the postmarks, he could follow their units' movements and pass on the intelligence to French agents. He was discovered in 1916 and had to sneak through German lines at Verdun. Marshal Philippe Pétain, then a hero, personally decorated him with the Légion d'Honneur.

My father was articulate and lively, winning friends with his warmth and intelligence. But then he became entangled in scientific controversy. Doctors had forbidden salt to nephritis patients. My father discovered that a lack of salt seriously increased urea in the blood. He was excluded by his colleagues, almost vilified, for revolutionary views. Later, when his hypothesis was proved correct, he was praised posthumously by those who had opposed his election to the Academy of Medicine.

The Rockefeller Foundation selected him to be among the first to use insulin, in 1922. His fame spread. I was conceived along the Nile, where my parents were honeymooning while he treated the king's diabetes.

My father loved research. At night, he visited young scientists and followed their progress. Nearly forty years later, I learned how this influenced my own career. At the time, Robert Courrier was experimenting with estrogen in rabbits. He was about to publish dramatic findings when my father brought him the *Journal of the American Medical Association*. Someone had beaten Courrier to it. Only in 1960, when he was permanent secretary of the Academy of Sciences, did I realize how Courrier had resented my father—and later his son—for bearing the bad news. He was among those who opposed my election to the Collège de France, where I would have been able to develop a course in reproduction, a very needed specialty in France at that time.

I know little about my father because my mother did not tell me much about him. She was his second wife, and he died in their fifth year together. An international lawyer, an English scholar, and a pianist, my mother was brilliant as well as beautiful. She traveled often to England where she championed the suffragettes. She felt hemmed in by Alsace and by my father's professional life. When he died, she broke all ties with his family. We moved to Paris, where I was allowed to think about any career I wanted. Except medicine.

My mother devoted herself to her three children's upbringing. We spent time with one of her brothers; the others were not deemed serious enough. The only weekend holiday of my childhood was a trip to Normandy with my uncle, where I discovered oysters.

The German Occupation made life dangerous for a single woman with children named Blum. We fled Paris for Grenoble, in the "free zone" not yet occupied by Hitler. In 1940, though still a boy, I was the only man in the family. With high school friends in a Communist-controlled group, I distributed anti-German tracts and broke windows of collaborators. The Gestapo took notice, and we moved away to the city of Annecy, in Haute-Savoie. There, I falsified my identification papers and became Emile Baulieu.

I was suddenly older on paper, to qualify for a tobacco ration card, but I was also growing up fast. My time was split between my studies and the French underground. When Haute-Savoie was liberated, I joined the army. At the end of 1944, I didn't know what to do. The Communist party wanted me to be a military officer or a party official. Instead, I followed a friend to medical school. Just to please my mother, I also enrolled in sciences.

Although I knew little about my father, I was drawn in his footsteps. It might have been a matter of genes. I would be a physician, with my father's fascination for science. Drifting from chemistry into biochemistry, I fell under the spell of Max-Fernand Jayle. He was a French original, a frail man who could hold a large hall in rapt attention.

Blinded young by an experiment with haptoglobin, a protein he discovered and then tracked all his life, Jayle seemed hardly aware of his handicap. With an assistant to help, he pressed on with his research and devoted hours to his students. Once, impressed with a seminar I had given, he asked what sort of career I wanted. Stuck for an answer, I said, "Like you." I became one of his. He took me into his family, offering warmth as well as knowledge.

After residency, I went back to Jayle. He got me a scholarship to study paper chromatography, a new technique from England, which started me on a double career, in the clinic and the laboratory. As a specialty, I chose hormones rather than haptoglobin; they were closer to my chemistry background and more immediately applicable to medicine. When Jayle was named chairman of the biochemistry department at the Faculté de Médecine in Paris, he made me a tenured professor. At thirty, I was freed of university politics.

I was also freed of politics in general. After Soviet tanks rolled into Hungary, I quit the party and threw myself totally into science. The best way to help society, I felt, was at the level of the individual. That was how doctors helped. My focus was summed up perfectly in a phrase by the Italian writer and chemist Primo Levi: "Science has an essential virtue. It respects what is."

Coming to New York, I had brought with me the baggage of a classically educated French scientist. My training was strict, within a system of masters and acolytes rooted deep in past centuries. The professor's word was almost scientific law, and his prejudices could reach far afield. I was a hybrid product coming from an old world and ready for a new outlook. Lieberman understood this well, joking about the system of "tin-hat dictators" from which he had borrowed me.

Years later, when I was inducted into the French Academy of Sciences, Lieberman was there to let the solemn gathering know in wry but respectful tones that science was part of the real world. Praising me, he was also describing himself: "Optimistic, enthusiastic, high-spirited, open-minded, cultured, serious, but always aware of the comedy, philosophic but never ponderous."

Working in New York, I could see up close all the often contradictory characteristics that gave the United States such leadership in science: the constant communication with others that was often tinged with excessive competition; the willingness to learn from abroad, mixed with national pride and an innate sense of superiority.

Lieberman and Pincus exemplified these contradictions, friendly rivals at the top of their field. While Lieberman was respected among his peers for avant-garde research, Pincus had a broad public following, a star-quality mystique, for his contraceptive pill. When Lieberman passed along Pincus's invitation for me to speak at the Worcester Foundation, near Boston, I was touched to note a certain nervousness. He gave me directions, and we set off, my wife, my three children, and me, in what was left of our $300 Ford.

When I finished my presentation, Pincus suggested that I stop off in Puerto Rico on my way home to talk with Dr. Celso Ramón García and his team, who were testing the new contraceptive pill. I was reluctant. It troubled me slightly that Hispanic women from a poor outlying territory were chosen for clinical trials (although the first human experiments had been done in Boston). I had no competence in contraception. Pincus urged me simply to take a look, and I thought I detected a twinkle in his eye.

As my plane lurched over the Caribbean, I was kicking

myself for this tropical escapade. Sick, a little afraid, I kept asking myself what I was doing there. But no sooner on the ground in San Juan, I saw the answer. One look at the clinical data suggested how the pill could change women's existence. From that Puerto Rican experience, I realized the impact on human life that the product of birth control research could have. I was hooked, although I didn't know it yet.

Pincus perfected his pill with John Rock, a staunch Catholic who taught gynecology and obstetrics at Harvard. Despite his faith, and in defiance of puritanical Boston society, Rock was of great help to his friend. He wrestled with his conscience, seeking to reconcile birth control with the Church's teachings. New England conservatives, bitterly opposed to the idea of an oral contraceptive, pressured him to abandon the research.

Rock was moved by a desire not only to help couples in their sexual lives but also to confront demographic waves which the world was beginning to notice. The election of Kennedy, a Catholic like himself, blunted the political conservatism of the preceding Eisenhower administration. Population control was in fashion again. Rock, convinced of the need to find a scientific breakthrough in contraception, organized clinical testing.

Rock wanted to monitor the release of the eggs, to reduce to a minimum the monthly abstinence required by the rhythm method—the only method sanctioned by Church authorities. Since any drug they developed to affect ovulation would amount to artificial means, Pincus and Rock knew they faced opposition. A third scientist weighed in, Min-Chueh Chang, an American biologist of Chinese origin. His experiments showed the effectiveness of taking synthetic progestins orally to block ovulation. At the beginning of the 1960s, this determined trio moved birth control from the mechanical to the medical.

Opponents, in the end, were no match for the prestige Pincus had built up over decades. Since 1944, he had edited a series of reports that summed up hormone research around the world. Private and government grants allowed him to expand his first small laboratory into the Worcester Foundation, not only a great research center but a source of inspiration for everyone in the field.

Before the war, Pincus had studied parthenogenesis, the division of the egg without fertilization by sperm. A Frenchman, Eugene Bataillon, had achieved this with sea urchins, by simply pricking the eggs. This produced only females, because the origin was a single female cell. What a revolution if women could produce women with no involvement from men! Pincus saw some initial promise with rabbits, but then abandoned the work.

It was later shown that parthenogenesis in mammals produces only primitive embryos, since growth seems to be blocked by the lack of male elements. But the simple fact that this is possible with invertebrates is vastly significant. It suggests the potential of a new individual arising in the absence of sexual reproduction.

Pincus also studied the stages of synthesis and breakdown of hormones and their role in certain mental disorders. In the early 1950s, his international role could hardly be matched. When he devoted himself to developing an oral contraceptive, I was disappointed. It seemed like a needless loss to pure science. But Pincus knew his idea's time had come.

The turning point came with Katharine Dexter McCormick, a socialite who had retired as a reclusive philanthropist when her young husband, Stanley, developed schizophrenia. Pincus was working on the hormonal biochemistry of psychiatric diseases, and this was one of those important but unpopular projects which Mrs. McCormick liked to support.

Mrs. McCormick told her friend Margaret Sanger about Pincus. Sanger, an ardent feminist and enlightened thinker, had resolved to put science in the service of women. She laid the groundwork for the Planned Parenthood Federation of America and its international affiliates. Condoms, withdrawal, or abstinence were not the answer to birth control, she knew. Diaphragms, which had to be fitted by specialists, were available only in a few modern clinics. Sanger arranged to meet with Pincus and Mrs. McCormick.

At that brief session, in 1951, Sanger convinced Pincus of

the need for a medical contraceptive that was easy for women to use. McCormick asked how much he would need for research. Pincus stalled; pressed again, he blurted out a number: $125,000. McCormick got out her checkbook. In the end, she gave almost $2 million to the Worcester Foundation.

At seventy, her fiery militancy cooling only slightly, Sanger whipped up support for Pincus. She could only spare $2,300 herself for Pincus's work, but she marshaled wealthy friends. The philanthropist Mary Lasker helped by setting up a prestigious award in this field, and she conferred the honor on Pincus.

The world was ready. "The pill" that Pincus began to speak about was no private quest of an endocrinologist who had spent too many hours in the laboratory. The idea had been floating around for decades. Aldous Huxley, the British novelist and philosopher, had looked in terror at the eventuality of humanity expanding out of control. In 1932, with no scientific basis, he wrote about a substance to control fertility in *Brave New World*. He called it "the pill."

Little research had been done before. In 1937, A. W. Makepeace and his collaborators at the University of Pennsylvania determined that a hormone, progesterone, could suspend ovulation. But they got no farther. Steroid hormones, synthesized by the body's glands, are secreted into the bloodstream without passing through the digestive tract. Taking a hormone orally rendered it ineffective. Scientists would have to find a derivative that would survive digestion. That was Pincus's starting point.

Carl Djerassi, who is still at work at Stanford University, had found the answer in 1949. He altered a molecule to synthesize a derivative, and Pincus knew "the pill" was possible.

Oral contraception works on the principle of daily absorption of a compound containing estrogen and a derivative of progesterone called progestin. Estrogen, like progesterone, is formed throughout pregnancy. Both work to block new ovulation during gestation. Until the placenta leaves the womb, no other eggs can be fertilized. Pincus's team determined the nature and quantity of hormones necessary to produce this same effect.

The pill is taken for three weeks, followed by a week to

allow bleeding, resembling menstruation, which cleanses the lining of the uterus and verifies contraception. Some women feel nauseous or bloated, but there are no lasting side effects. If the pill is not resumed, the woman's physiology returns to normal.

Now widely used, this method faced a storm of objections equal to the fury over RU-486 twenty-five years later. Rumors circulated that it could be dangerous over a long period. Antoine Lacassagne, one of the great scientists of his age, had shown that prolonged exposure to estrogens could produce breast cancer in some strains of mice. Despite overwhelming scientific evidence that this specific situation did not apply generally, the specter of cancer was raised.

Another specter, sterility, was also trotted out. Women on the pill were described as "temporarily sterile," with the word meant to shock. This, of course, was ridiculous. In fact, women cannot conceive except around the time of ovulation. And ovulation suspended by the pill resumed as soon as the woman stopped taking it. Some detractors, with a tinge of racism, felt that the pill's tests in San Juan proved nothing for women of the developed world.

Allan Parkes, a celebrated physiologist, dismissed critics with his wry British wit: "No woman should be kept on the Pill for twenty years until, in fact, a sufficient number have been kept on the Pill for twenty years."

The critics were wrong. There have been some ill effects in women over the past thirty years, and there will likely be others. But they are negligible compared with the number of healthy women who have been able to control their fertility and spare themselves the hardship of unwanted pregnancies. This is especially true in the Third World, where childbearing amounts to a serious health risk for so many women.

The pill, whatever one's own ideological position on its use, has spared countless lives. It has made many more lives richer and safer. Improvements in its formulation have reduced some of its early discomfort. Aside from its role in family planning, it has decreased the number of ovarian and endometrial cancers and benign breast tumors.

Young women today can hardly imagine the courage and

perseverance it took to put into practice this modern form of birth control. A woman knows that the choice is hers. But it would be a far different story if Pincus and his colleagues had simply published their findings on animals and suggested that the method was promising for humans whenever someone wanted to try it.

Happily, their work found a resounding echo among others who made it their mission to speak out on behalf of women. Science joined with society, and both moved forward. Now, women take for granted the freedom of choice allowed by the pill, just as we no longer marvel at images on a television screen.

But for the first time on a broad scale, sexuality had been separated from its reproductive consequences. The pill was a medical revolution. Even more, by setting women free in a larger sense, it changed the world forever.

Back in Paris, though fascinated by the Pincus pill, I resumed my own work. Thanks to Lieberman, I was a confirmed professional, able to set a clear course and follow it with the best means available. He and I were the only ones who were systematically studying dehydroepiandrosterone sulfate. This posed a financial problem, however.

To progress, I would need to buy radioactive hormones and expensive instruments to handle them. In the past, Jayle had found funds for me in his budget at the Ecole de Puériculture, where he ran a clinical chemistry laboratory for measuring hormones in pregnant women. Now he was beginning to worry that my research was encroaching on his territory, straining our warm relationship. And his own resources were limited.

A stroke of luck made the difference. Recent reforms made it possible, finally, for a French scientist to pursue a decently paid career at a university hospital without maintaining a private practice. With fresh blood, and a small flood of francs, the old National Health Institutes was converted into INSERM. The directors decided to jump a generation and offer opportunities to younger researchers. It was a bold step, breaking for the first time with the rigid system of hierarchy.

My name was put forward. Without even asking, I found myself at the head of an independent INSERM research unit with technicians, a secretary, and the means to take in students and foreign scientists. It was Research Unit 33, the same "U-33" I direct today. Its high technology is housed in a new building at Bicêtre Hospital, originally a thirteenth-century fort, and my office overlooks the former insane asylum where the Marquis de Sade was kept for some time during the French Revolution. The name *Unité 33, trente-trois,* was a pleasing touch. Generations of French doctors have examined patients' chest cavities by asking them to say *"trente-trois."*

That was my turning point. It was also my only option. Just as Professor Courrier's secret blackball had veered me away from a career at the Collège de France, political infighting had closed another important door for me. I had been invited to work at a medical unit under Lucien de Gennes, a brilliant endocrine specialist, and perhaps succeed him as chief of medicine at Broussais Hospital. Hostility among some of his colleagues blocked my appointment, however. It turned out to be another fortunate stroke of fate. At the hospital, my first responsibility would have been to patients. It would have been a rewarding career, but at the expense of my research.

Pincus kept in touch. In 1964, he asked me to talk about my work at one of his famed scientific gatherings, that year at Lake George in upstate New York. We stayed in small chalets by the water; Pincus and his wife were in a larger one in our midst. I have forgotten the discussion about my paper, but I can still see the great doctor and his wife sweeping into the dining room, he in black tie and she in a shimmering lamé evening dress. With true Old World decorum, we had all dressed for dinner.

Afterward, Pincus offered his help. He named me to an international committee that organized world congresses on steroid hormones. He put me on a WHO panel of experts that met regularly in Geneva to consider population and reproduction problems. He was charming and offhand, but his goal was clear enough. He wanted a circle of specialists who could advance his most beloved project: to develop methods of contraception.

Hormone research was a relatively small field. Friendships came fast, but competitiveness could take strange forms. After my Lake George talk, I walked out to the pool and found a man with myopic eyes and a large balding head sitting on the edge, dunking his feet. It was Oscar Hechter, coauthor with Pincus of the classic work on the synthesis of adrenal hormones. He saw himself as the central theoretician of hormone biology and would have liked to influence research globally. A little nervous, I asked what he had thought of my presentation.

He wasn't there, he said, with harsh rudeness. What's more, dehydroepiandrosterone sulfate and hormone metabolism were of no interest to anyone. I backed away with a frozen smile and stayed bitter for years. It was only when we met again at Pincus's funeral, and after he spent a year in my lab on a sabbatical leave, that I understood his reaction. It was frustration.

Hechter knew that a man of his drive and intelligence could have gone farther. His original work and observant analysis had added much to the field of hormones. Eventually, we got to be close friends, and his advice helped me in preparing this book.

On returning from my year in New York, in 1962, I received a call from Jean-Claude Roussel, president of Roussel-Uclaf, then the second largest pharmaceutical company in France. Friends had spoken to him about me. He was lively and likable, with a warm, generous charm. His staunch conservatism did not dim an adventuresome spirit in areas beyond politics. His father had built the family business and, before dying, asked that it not be sold. Jean-Claude might have been rich and carefree; he loved hunting, sports cars, aircraft, and grand trips abroad. But he had studied pharmacy and felt bound to carry on the Roussel name.

I was no great admirer of the pharmaceutical industry. It seemed to me like a mercantile deviation of scientific research. I've since changed my mind. In countries with no private drug companies, patients suffer the consequences. The Soviet Union, for example, is desperately short of contraceptives; its abortion rate is several times its birth rate, the reverse of the United States and France.

A university laboratory can concentrate only on one or two subjects, with no immediate need to put findings to use. The pharmaceutical industry cannot afford knowledge for its own sake. It must focus on compounds that are not only effective but marketable and profitable as well. Its researchers must balance pure science against conflicting interests that touch on finance, politics, ethics, and personal ambitions.

Roussel asked if I would take over as head of research. He hardly knew me but must have trusted his instincts. My immediate refusal surprised him. Academic freedom had more value than corporate power and money, and I was happy doing public research. Instead, we designed my post of a consultant. In exchange for suggestions given exclusively to Roussel-Uclaf, I could test some of my hypotheses in large, high-quality laboratories and receive for my work at INSERM compounds otherwise difficult to obtain.

The arrangement raised some eyebrows. Back then, the line was sacrosanct between academic scientists and those who turned science into profit. In our hallowed halls, moving to private industry was a demeaning sellout. There was also a whiff of envy; private industry paid far higher salaries. But the principles were firm. If free-enterprise competition spurred quality, no private group should benefit unfairly; scientific advances belonged to all of society. Practical application did not necessarily have to follow discovery. Science was sacred; business was profane.

It was a matter of balance. Academics were right to preserve their independence and their traditions. But more cross-feeding was essential. Over the years the gulf has narrowed between those scientists who break ground in pure isolation and those who must carry it on to the people who will benefit. For me, this gulf is still too wide.

My association with Roussel-Uclaf was fruitful from the beginning, on both sides. After Jean-Claude Roussel was killed in a helicopter accident in 1972, I found myself drawn even closer to the possibilities of working with the company. Edouard Sakiz, my old colleague and kindred spirit, took over as president.

* * *

By 1965, I realized that, for the time being, I had done about all I could with dehydroepiandrosterone sulfate. Although I had discovered how to trace its secretion, I did not know much about its effect in the human body. That was a whole new area, and I lacked the clinical facilities to explore it. In any case, it was time to move on. I had seen too many lab directors base their existence on a single discovery at the beginning of their career. It was better to branch out and come back later with a fresh approach.

In looking for a new challenge, I wanted to take advantage of my steroid experience. It was the right time to start looking at hormones in a different way. Molecular biology had studied microbes and viruses, but it had not been applied to animal science. A new biology was taking shape, and I wanted to be a part of it—and use it in hormone research.

It was only in 1963, after James Watson and Francis Crick won a Nobel Prize for their work on DNA, that most of us realized the importance of studying the molecular makeup beneath the maladies that captivated medical science. Their brilliantly simple explanations shone light down paths we had ignored. Looking around, I found only a few trailblazers.

Elwood Jensen at the Ben May Laboratory in Chicago had devised a way to mark an estradiol derivative with radioactive tritium, which allowed him to track the hormone. His discovery, that this estrogen remained in the uterus rather than other organs, took research forward. The strategy was simple but revolutionary: look at where a hormone goes instead of what it does.

We knew a lot about the regulatory action of hormones: how they triggered changes when added or subtracted. We knew they were signal mechanisms which tell the body to respond in specific ways. The more abundant they are, the stronger action they trigger. Still, we did not know all the components. In the mid-1960s, medicine was responding in the classic nineteenth-century manner: surgeons removed glands to reduce hormones. Instead, I was after ways to tamper with the signals.

By finding—and blocking—the specific receptor molecules, scientists could operate at the level of the target cells. It would not matter whether hormone flows were decreased. The same amount could remain in the body if their messages were not delivered. A new endocrinology was developing, based on the action of receptors. The key, obviously, was to study these receptors.

Following Jensen, a great deal of work had been done on the estrogen receptor. I focused my laboratory's attention on this and other sex steroid receptors. The need for more research in that area was obvious. Any discoveries would advance the science of birth control. Pincus's enthusiasm had infected me, and I wanted to keep working in the directions pioneered by his work. Where Pincus had worked in physiology, we could now do molecular endocrinology.

At that time, birth control in France was virtually unexplored territory. I kept up with international developments, through Pincus and the WHO meetings in Geneva. Soon, my work in science spilled over into politics.

Under a 1920 law, Frenchwomen were banned from using any contraceptive methods. Only condoms were available, tolerated officially but quietly to prevent diseases from prostitutes. Neither the diaphragm nor the newly developed IUD was legal. François Mitterrand made abolition of this archaic law part of his campaign for the presidency in 1965. He lost the election, but the idea remained. The health minister named a committee of thirteen "wise men," including myself, to study the question.

Only two of us had any notion of what was happening abroad. No one had any direct medical experience with the forbidden pill but, with some reserve, we voted for it. Our detailed report was kept confidential, pending government decision, but the next week *Paris Match* produced a cover showing a contented mother, smiling and serene, with a baby in her arms. The headline read, "Green Light for the Pill." It was a perfect illustration of our position: women with a choice were happier mothers. I was known for my pro-pill position, and I supplied most of the data to the committee. Opponents accused me of leaking our views to build public support. Not so. I don't know who leaked them, but France rallied around. Shortly after Charles de Gaulle was elected, the National Assembly voted for permitting contraception in France.

At INSERM, we worked long hours on steroid receptors.

Young researchers from Roussel-Uclaf came by, learning from us and preparing the technology for pharmaceutical applications of our studies. At the same time, I was understanding more about the world in which my experiments might play a part. At the Geneva meetings, I was steeped in reports citing the desperation over the lack of contraception in poor countries. I dreamed of developing new methods with original research in my own laboratory.

In 1970, I took time out to travel to India with a delegation of French intellectuals who wanted to see the Third World situation firsthand. Bombay, Calcutta, and Benares brought to life those graphs of demographic figures I had seen so often in Geneva.

One morning, stepping into the human wave flowing across the bridge by Calcutta's railroad station, I was jostled and pushed along by people fighting for the space to move forward. Beggars lined the railings, each competing desperately for the limited sympathy of hard-pressed passersby. One woman thrust the corpse of a baby in my face. "Touch it, you'll see he is dead," she implored. "You see! Give me money."

During that trip, I decided to aim my life's work toward finding some way to ease this sort of suffering. It is a common enough goal for conscientious Westerners when they see the Third World up close. But I felt I was unusually placed to make a contribution with impact. At the same time, when we met Indira Gandhi, I realized that the answer did not lie in the calm confines of science alone.

When I proposed work on a once-a-week pill, Mrs. Gandhi flashed her fierce nationalism and replied, "Why not an Indian pill?" It was an inappropriate reaction. But she differed from many Third World leaders who saw a bigger challenge in raising the stature of their societies than in keeping them to a manageable size. Some encouraged childbirth so that their countries would have the clout of a higher census.

Political and social obstacles were inescapable, not only in developing countries but everywhere else. In France, they were formidable. With a new birth control law in effect, France had to organize research, train specialists, and institute the surveillance of oral contraceptives. The government funded a joint program to combine these concerns with the study of embryonic development and infant diseases. But research in birth control lagged far behind. Something beyond matters of money and the competence of specialists dampened French research in this crucial new field. It was ironic, since Frenchwomen became among the most frequent users of the pill. The problem, perhaps, was the cultural and educational background of our doctors and researchers—a reflection of the larger society. Contraception is much practiced in France, but not often openly discussed, not even by influential women.

I had found this strange reticence in my work with Roussel-Uclaf. Late in the 1960s, Sakiz, then chief of a research laboratory at Romainville, and I proposed a pill to block ovulation, à la Pincus. It would have been safer and better tolerated than any yet available, using new progestin steroids synthesized by Roussel chemists. It promised commercial success, in France and beyond. The project was pursued reluctantly and marketed with little enthusiasm, leaving the field to Schering, in Berlin, and Organon, a Dutch company, which shared the market with the Americans.

This setback reflected a larger failing. The French could not grasp the importance of population problems. The resistance came from the top levels of government back then and, for the most part, still comes from these same quarters today. France provides no funds to WHO programs in this field. Frenchmen prefer loftier concepts, such as geopolitics and ecology, to demography. Only Jacques Cousteau has tried recently to make people aware of the issue. There is a deeply rooted ambiguity in our culture, our mentality, in regard to birth control.

RU-486 came about like many scientific discoveries. One step followed another, and another, and then the next step went off in a different direction entirely. In science, the shortest distance between two points can be a long detour.

I chose the direction of sex hormones and their receptors

despite some advice to turn elsewhere. All steroids share common properties, and my work might have been more successful in the field of cortisones. These are used widely in medicine and bring a high return to pharmaceutical companies. But Pincus had kindled my desire to contribute to fertility control, one way or another.

The first steps toward RU-486 were taken in the mid-1960s when I assembled my research team at U-33 to begin tracking hormones to their receptors. The Ford Foundation gave us a long-term grant of $750,000 and, at my insistence, left it free of strings. The Ford funds were earmarked for population control, but I wanted freedom for research to range widely. I knew my work would eventually end up where Ford wanted it to go. But I felt I first had to understand the mechanisms of sex hormones, and also, if possible, contribute to another medical field. In fact, our research was diverse during the fifteen years it took us to develop RU-486. Those identified with noted discoveries are never wholly focused on one area, and often many people are involved, one way or another. Indeed, diversification may contribute most to the success of a specific discovery. We proceed with open minds.

Steroid hormone receptors are so few in the body that they defied available chemical methods to study them in detail. At the beginning, we looked for more accessible proteins which also bound to steroids. We identified a likely protein in the blood which we called SBP, for sex steroid binding plasma protein (it is also known as SHBG, for sex hormone binding globulin, and is frequently assayed in medical practice). But its binding characteristics were completely different from those of receptors. While receptors mediate the action of hormones, this sort of protein only transports them. We needed a more direct approach.

We perfected systems for measuring receptors. Henri Rochefort, then a resident, logged several important observations on the estradiol receptor before moving on with his own career. Now a professor of molecular biology at Montpellier, he is one of the world's leading experts on breast cancer.

To advance, we had to look at other sex hormones. We

made some discoveries about testosterone which helped form the basis for the treatment of prostatic tumors. Then a friend of Rochefort's, Edwin Milgrom, also a talented physician and scientist, joined the laboratory to help us zero in on the progesterone receptor.

We first tried Elwood Jensen's method of tracing radioactive progestin to a target, in this case the uterus of a laboratory rat. Results were limited because, we learned later, receptors in the rat are particularly fragile. We had more success with the technique we used in studying the estrogen receptor; we ground up a uterus and examined the binding of the progesterone hormone to the receptor in a test tube. This worked best with guinea pigs, which, like women, have a twenty-eight-day cycle.

Edwin and I observed that we could find more of the progesterone receptors by first injecting laboratory animals with estradiol, the natural estrogen, simulating what occurs during the first part of a woman's cycle. This demonstrated a basic principle of hormone physiology: one hormone, estradiol, can facilitate the action of a second hormone, progesterone, by augmenting its receptors.

By 1969, we had tracked down the progesterone receptor in the uterus of a guinea pig. Looking back, that was a significant step toward developing RU-486. At the time, however, it was only an experiment with radioactive progestin. We still had to learn whether a steroid that binds to the progesterone receptor has to be a progestin, which mimics progesterone action, or if it could be an antagonist, which blocks progesterone action. We had found the receptor, but we still were looking for an antagonist steroid, and we had to determine whether it would bind to the receptor we had identified.

While we worked at solving the puzzle in our own laboratory, I kept in close contact with distant colleagues, and I looked in other directions. A scientific researcher, unlike a bulldozer driver, cannot plow forward in a single line after a specific objective. He must attack the whole mountain, with a few objectives in mind. Eventually, he may uncover what he is looking for. He may also find something else.

After tracing the progesterone receptor, I took our early findings to the United States to confer with Bert O'Malley, whose research team at NIH was studying the role of hormones in egg production in chickens. We were at once colleagues and competitors in that curious manner of researchers probing similar ground. The findings of one could help the other, but differing points of view had led us off in separate directions. I warned O'Malley about the mistake we had made with a blood protein; we had learned that this compound could mimic the binding of hormones to the receptors and falsify results.

In 1970, scientists gathered for the first international meeting on receptors, which I organized in Berlin. Our observations were confirmed: we were breaking new ground, but we also learned others were doing important work in related areas.

Once detected, progesterone receptors were easy enough to study. In my laboratory we noted that not only did they increase in number when we administered estrogen but also that they decreased when confronted with progesterone. This is an effect known as down regulation. Once the progesterone delivered its message, the concentration of receptors diminished; it was a natural defense against excessive action from the hormone.

This negative effect of progesterone on its receptor pointed me to a new principle applicable to the problems posed by human fertility. I knew I was onto something important. If we could decrease the activity of progesterone receptors with a drug and prevent the effect of the hormone, we could temporarily alter the reproductive process. That is the crux of birth control.

We tried out a "midcycle" pill, a compound designated as RU-2323, which could decrease the progesterone receptor without displaying any progesterone activity. It showed promise of preventing pregnancy by taking pills only once a week, substantially reducing the discomfort many women felt with twenty-one-day doses of hormones.

Tests in Haiti were not convincing enough, however, and we moved on. It was hardly time wasted. By 1975, the principle of a method to reduce progesterone activity was clearly on my mind, but the paper I published on that subject, "Antiprogesterone Effect and Midcycle (Periovulapory) Contraception," hardly provoked a reaction.

We were able to intensify our research by isolating receptors and obtaining antibodies. Hélène Richard-Foy devised new techniques, and Linda Fox, an American student, turned up the first antireceptor antibodies. We improved our methods and Michel Renoir came out ahead in our years-old dispute with O'Malley's team, now in Houston, over the isolation of the progesterone receptor. In my laboratory, Jean-Marie Gasc, of the Collège de France, perfected a way to follow the progesterone receptor with a microscope. He showed that it is situated in the nucleus of the receptor cell, even in the absence of hormones.

From the beginning of my research, I took interest in work by Jack Gorski at the University of Illinois. He had determined that receptors in body tissue not yet exposed to hormones were large, inactive molecules. Once they bound with hormones, these large receptors were transformed into smaller, active forms to adhere to the genes they regulate.

I felt it would be easier to isolate these larger receptors, but it took some effort to convince my colleagues. Jan Mester, a young Slovak chemist who did not want to return to his country after the calamitous Prague Spring of 1968, energized this phase of the research. I had met him in London and took him back to Paris, where he eventually settled as a French citizen.

Once we began working with the large receptors, results came fast, and our field of study widened. I worked for years with Maria-Grazia Catelli, an Italian gynecologist who had taken up molecular biology, to probe into complex protein interaction. We saw that the receptor molecule's structure was heterogeneous; it contained not only the progesterone receptor but also another protein, a "heat-shock protein" (hsp), which did not bind the hormone.

When cells are aggravated by stress or fever, they react by producing heat-shock proteins. These help other protein components to modify their shape so that cells can resist the shock. We found that in the absence of a hormone, an hsp acts as a cap on the receptor which prevents it from interacting with genes.

After a hormone binds to it, the receptor changes its shape and shucks off the hsp. Uncapped, the receptor makes contact with the DNA of genes and delivers its message.

By 1975, we had yet to find a molecule that bound to the progesterone receptor and countered hormonal action. We kept looking, but I decided to shift my sights.

Who knows why a researcher suddenly changes course? It may be the simple tedium of frequenting the same molecules, the same specialists, with microscopic familiarity. There is the element of renewing a quest by reexamining the old questions from another angle. For whatever reason, a fortunate encounter turned me in a new direction: the action of steroids on the surface of cells.

At a lecture, I learned that progesterone triggers the division of the egg, the process of meiosis, at least in amphibians. About that time, Sabine Schorderet-Slatkine called me from the University of Geneva. She had gone far in the study of meiosis but had searched in vain for a progesterone receptor in the cell membrane. I assumed she was using the wrong techniques, and I suggested that we combine forces.

Preliminary work showed that Sabine was right. We were not seeing what was normally expected, a receptor in the nucleus of the cell. Over several rigorous, passionate years of research, we found a new type of progesterone receptor, different from the one I knew. It was situated in the external membrane of the cell, and did not act on the genes. The discovery opened up a new range of steroid research.

It seemed as if thwarting meiosis might produce a new type of contraception action. By blocking the new type of progesterone receptor in the cell membrane, we could prevent the egg from ripening enough to be fertilized. But the study of meiosis was difficult in mammals; contrary to what happens with amphibians, it is not triggered by a hormone. It would be hard to do the fundamental research, and we were far from any new contraceptive. I left the project hanging rather than wander off too far in an area beyond my competence. But isolating this new receptor raised some other intriguing questions.

If we had found membrane receptors in a certain type of cell, where else might we find them? A likely candidate was the central nervous system, where electric phenomena depend on changes in the cell membranes and occur quickly. This broad hypothesis rekindled my earlier fascination with the central nervous system, back when I was a resident in psychiatry at Salpêtrière Hospital in Paris.

I had some clues. Colette Corpéchot, a research technician studying dehydroepiandrosterone sulfate since the early days of my research, had detected that compound in the brain tissue of rats, curiously enough, since it is not secreted by adrenal glands in these animals as it is in primates. The steroid had to originate in the rat's nervous system itself. We rechecked the data, and Jan Sjovall of the Karolinska Institute in Stockholm confirmed the observation by examining our extracts with mass spectrometry. I called this type of steroid a "neurosteroid."

Paul Robel, my perennial, indispensable associate, and a group of young researchers helped me, but we moved slowly. We were not trained neurobiologists. Still, those early results suggested significant discoveries to be made in the central nervous system. Indeed, certain neurosteroids modulate the effect of one of the receptors of GABA (gamma-aminobutyric acid), a neurotransmitter that calms nerve function.

These first meanderings captivated me, opening fresh fields for research that would come later.

Another apparent detour in research, toward chickens, turned out to be an important step toward RU-486. This was also in the mid-1970s, and originally it was a welcome venture into pure research.

As a biological model for a precise biochemical analysis of steroid hormones, we chose the synthesis of proteins in chicken egg white. The huge capacity of oviducts to synthesize these proteins simplified our experiments. We could administer hormones and antihormones and easily watch their activity.

Robert Sutherland, a New Zealander who had studied in Australia came to INSERM and worked on tamoxifen, an antiestrogen used to treat breast cancer. Sutherland demonstrated that this powerful substance acted forcefully in chickens as a pure antiestrogen, with no estrogen effect, contrary to what occurs in women. Tamoxifen fights breast cancers linked to estrogens by blocking the hormone's action. This was the effect we wanted to have on progesterone.

I was struck by the chemistry of tamoxifen relating to its antihormone activity. Its molecular structure resembled diethylstilbestrol, or DES, a potent synthetic estrogen. The difference was an additional chemical cycle grafted onto the molecule, which turned an estrogen into an antiestrogen. The idea of finding an antagonistic structural analog of progesterone as different from that hormone as tamoxifen is different from DES, in fact, has nothing to do with DES activity. This has never been understood by the blind opponents of RU-486.

In the 1950s two American doctors, in the mistaken belief that a lack of estrogen caused spontaneous abortions, gave large doses of DES to women in danger of miscarrying. A few years later, most daughters of these patients showed abnormalities of the genital tract; about 1 percent of them had cancerous tumors. The molecule DES was not to blame as such. The error was in giving a strong estrogen while an embryo was developing. In fact, DES was the first drug used successfully against cancer—in Chicago in the 1940s, by Nobel laureate Charles Huggins.

The unusual makeup of the tamoxifen molecule gave me an important clue. It had the same basic structure as DES. And the antihormonal chemical cycle grafted onto it did not prevent its binding to the estrogen receptor, just as DES did. Clearly, the "keyhole" in hormone receptors allowed a certain leeway. It might be possible to graft some sort of chemical cycle onto other hormones, like progestins, to make the antihormone we were seeking.

I relayed my optimism to Robert Bucourt, chief chemist at Roussel-Uclaf, and some of the company's senior pharmacologists. We had promising ground for lab work.

This passing connection to diethylstilbestrol, slight as it was, would haunt us later on. Opponents of RU-486 called it a "chemical time bomb" because it might repeat damage done by DES;

the mere mention of DES is enough to strike fear. Scientifically, that is ridiculous. RU-486 has no relation to DES.

Throughout the 1970s, as we pushed ahead on the road toward an antiprogesterone, I was involved in several lines of research not directly related to fertility control. I believe that keeping other irons in the fire stimulates a laboratory, intellectually as well as technically, and therefore enhances its potential for other options.

At U-33, I am responsible for the futures of all the researchers on its team. In this little collection of different personalities and interests, each must find a niche. Students are just starting their careers. Older scientists are reshaping theirs. The human part is enjoyable, with its constant intellectual interplay. The scientific part is challenging, pursuing separate parts toward a whole. In this setting, the chance of an unexpected discovery comes in the context of an overall coherent strategy.

Roussel-Uclaf was a help to us, but its priorities were different. Even if I had had a clearer view of where we were going toward an antiprogesterone, I could not have told Roussel. In the trade, sex hormones had a dubious reputation. Their commercial potential was regarded as limited, and pharmaceutical companies adhere to the same bottom line as every other business.

The company had given only tepid backing to the oral contraceptive we had proposed in 1968. Its directors were not anxious to go farther during the 1970s. They felt that the field was already amply covered, and few of them would be prepared to invest in an abortion pill.

This view, in fact, was widely held around the world. After ten years on the market, the oral contraceptive had proven itself to be effective and fairly well tolerated. It was expected to be increasingly accepted and distributed in the Third World. To improve on the pill's principle, scientists were working on injectable or implantable hormone preparations capable of stopping ovulation for months at a time. Several types of IUD had been perfected; a single device could protect a woman for years, offering an alternative to those who suffered side effects from the hormonal methods. There was also sterilization.

At first glance, the figures seemed to show that birth control was being practiced more and more. In all, more than 120 million women and more than 50 million men had been sterilized. Another 70 million women used an IUD. And each year about 50 million used the pill. The logical assumption was that the number of abortions would rapidly drop. But that was not the case.

Seen from another perspective, the numbers were unsettling. Sterilization amounted to mutilation, and I did not like its irreversibility. No other method was reliable enough. For all the pill's promise, only about 5 percent of fertile women were using it. Women did not always take it regularly; its failure rate surpassed 15 percent in some places.

Among the few specialists who sounded the alarm, Lidija Andolsek of Yugoslavia was especially moving. At a WHO session in Geneva, her testimony on the grave consequences of abortion rang out, with cool passion. Most of us were men and could not have the same perception. She had her facts, and she drove home what they meant. Her plea convinced me that even if contraceptive methods were an important step, they were not enough.

If the number of abortions had dipped in some developed countries, it was soaring in parts of the Third World and in the Soviet bloc countries, where contraceptives were scarce. Where abortions were illegal, or where legal ones were hard to obtain, women continued to suffer and die.

If reality moved drug company executives as humans, it promised little for the profit-and-loss statement. Too many questions about antiprogesterones remained unsolved. After finding the progesterone receptor, we still had no antiprogestin that would bind to it effectively. We had had a glimmer of hope with RU-2323, but it let us down. There was no compound capable of orienting chemical research toward our goal.

Scientists were not even sure that the effect of an antiprogesterone on animals was applicable to humans. Although progesterone seemed indispensable during gestation for rats and rabbits, nothing proved that an antiprogesterone could stop pregnancy in a woman.

The last word had not been spoken on controlling human fertility. We were all beginning to see the need for new techniques adapted to different conditions of life, according to country, culture, age, and family situation. The methods available did not cover all the needs, and they were proving less effective than we had believed.

Abortion was a medical problem that would not soon disappear. Women in every society, from the most advanced to the least developed, badly needed an easier but extremely effective way to approach birth control. For some, happiness and self-fulfillment were in the balance. For many others, the stakes were higher.

A new hope surfaced with prostaglandins. In Sweden, Bergström, Samuelsson, and Bygdeman had designed a study program on second-trimester abortions, with clinical work at Karolinska Hospital. I went to Stockholm several times for WHO to evaluate the work for research support. None of us knew then how closely our separate but parallel paths would merge a few years later.

The line of inquiry was firing imaginations. In 1970, Carl Djerassi published in *Science* magazine an article entitled "Birth Control After 1984," evoking the Orwellian vision of life under Big Brother. Djerassi's predictions held up better than George Orwell's. He foresaw a compound to halt the cycle and stop pregnancy at its beginning. Ideally, he wrote, this would work at any time during the first eight weeks. Strangely, he did not mention an antiprogesterone. He suggested instead a process of luteolysis, the regression of the corpus luteum, to drop the progesterone level. And he thought this would be possible with prostaglandins, already studied in domestic animals.

Unfortunately, no one ever came up with a compound, natural or synthetic, that worked well enough on the corpus luteum in humans. Prostaglandins would eventually prove to be effective in stopping pregnancy, mainly because of the way they stimulate the uterine muscle and dilate the cervix. But they also provoked strong contractions of the digestive organs, which could cause nausea, vomiting, diarrhea, and sometimes cardiovascular troubles. Researchers would later find derivatives with fewer side effects, especially those administered locally or orally.

My own interest in antihormones for birth control grew steadily, piqued by accounts of suffering in the Third World. Each day, five hundred women died from botched abortions. And three times that many died from the complications of pregnancy. The progress made in developed countries had little impact in many countries because of poor nutrition and hygiene, inadequate medical facilities, or social and cultural conditions.

Although my brief venture toward a midcycle pill, with RU-2323, had been disappointing, it delineated the territory. It seemed nearly impossible to base a practical method of contraception on cyclical hormonal changes. Even among the most regular women, timing can shift significantly from one month to the next. I pressed onward, seeking other possibilities.

In 1976, WHO gave me a small grant to study progesterone receptors in the uterus during the cycle and at the beginning of pregnancy. We had shown how hormones affect the concentration of receptors in the guinea pig uterus, but it was time to make the vital jump to humans. In examining biopsies of the uterine lining, the endometrium, provided by Créteil Hospital near Paris, we found similar variations. It was tempting to extrapolate the results toward broader conclusions.

I was finally convinced that progesterone had to be my prime target when I learned of the work of Arpad Csapo, a Hungarian-born biochemist in St. Louis. He proved that progesterone was indispensable to the start of pregnancy, making it clear to me that an antiprogestin would produce the opposite effect: miscarriage, or abortion. Csapo's results were confirmed by studies of uterine fragments, which suggested how effectively progesterone calms uterine contractions. He showed how the hormone counteracts the abortive effect of prostaglandins.

Csapo also demonstrated in animals that even a very brief interruption of progesterone's effect causes irreversible changes in the endometrium that prevent implantation, thus causing abortion.

No doubt remained. Physiological studies and work on receptors had clearly defined the role of progesterone and its mechanisms. Science had advanced, but the needs remained. By the end of the 1970s, I was disappointed by results from family planning centers supported by WHO. No new method of fertility control was in sight.

In a number of countries, skillful teams were working with the latest techniques. But there was resistance, the perennial controversy surrounding any method of birth control. Limiting procreation is different from working with sick people who take medication without a thought to its deeper meaning. Birth control involves people in good health, with personal and cultural considerations of family as well as their own bodies.

WHO's initial ardor had begun to cool. Research on contraception had diminished in university laboratories around the world. It was all but nonexistent in the pharmaceutical industry. And yet statistics revealed the desperately high level of abortions.

My own goal was clear. An antiprogesterone compound could almost certainly provide a medical alternative that was less traumatizing than other methods in use. I had changed a great deal from my first days with Pincus and my meanderings in a general direction. I was after something specific.

My association with Roussel-Uclaf was crucial to finding the right compound. Biologists might find a purpose for synthesizing new molecules, but chemists must actually make them. For any pharmaceutical company, its wealth is in its own chemistry. Drugs can be made with compounds patented by others, but profits must then be shared. Like most of the glory, most of the earnings come from original laboratory work. Leaders in the industry are largely chemists; Edouard Sakiz is a rare exception. Roussel-Uclaf's laboratories were widely known for their fine chemistry, especially with steroids.

But changes were afoot. In 1976, the company named Jacques Boissier as head of research. A well-known pharmacologist and a powerful university professor, he was a specialist in the central nervous system and had no interest in hormones. He knew that drugs based on steroids, as opposed to, say, antibiotics, earned little. And once he shifted to private industry, he insisted that all research lead toward profit.

Apparently neither Boissier nor other senior people I had briefed at Roussel-Uclaf passed on to laboratory chemists my observations about the structure of tamoxifen and its potential for synthesizing other receptor-binding compounds.

Fortunately for my purposes, progesterone is closely related to cortisone and its derivatives. Cortisone pays its way. Together with its derivatives, it can control metabolism, blood pressure levels, and some nervous system functions. It can affect certain tumors, and acts on infections, inflammation, allergies, shock, stress, burns, and wounds.

Antiglucocorticosteroids, which counteract the activity of cortisone and cortisone-like hormones, had not been applied to any particular disorder, because none had yet been developed for use. Research in that direction would be useful, at the same time, in looking for an antiprogesterone. Some specialists doubted the medical value of a cortisone antagonist. To simplify research and to pursue well-defined results, I suggested work on an antiglucocorticosteroid to speed the healing of burns and wounds, as well as the treatment of glaucoma. This would be relatively easy to test, since the product would be given locally and would probably be free of side effects. Also, it would be free of controversy.

At annual meetings between managers and researchers, my speeches stirred little enthusiasm or comment. But everyone agreed that we should devote at least some resources to steroids, and few wanted to deprive Roussel-Uclaf of high-quality research. Happily, the company maintained its capacity for chemical study of hormones and antihormones.

Two representatives from Hoechst sat in on the meetings, silently keeping an eye on the bottom line. But I also had a pair of allies, two consultants like myself. Edouard Housset, who became dean of the medical school at Broussais-Hôtel-Dieu hospital, insisted on the medical potential of steroid research. And Derek Barton fell with a vengeance on the slightest scientific imprecision that might arise in discussions. Sir Derek, a chemist and a true genius, lent considerable weight to my arguments.

Mostly, it was support from Sakiz that kept my proposals from being shelved in favor of something more obviously lucrative. As a former hormone researcher of great talent, he understood the importance of our work. As company president, he had enough influence to ensure at least grudging support for endocrinology. That was all we needed.

Georges Teutsch, one of those chemists behind Roussel-Uclaf's reputation, synthesized RU-486 in 1980. He followed a course of research that I had also charted. The molecule was what Roussel-Uclaf wanted, an antiglucocorticosteroid. And although neither Teutsch nor most of the others in the company initially realized it, it was also what I wanted: an antiprogesterone. Under the circumstances, it is amazing to see how such a versatile molecule might emerge in research.

The irony was brought home in a letter Teutsch wrote me when a journalist reported that Teutsch felt he should be regarded as the father of RU-486. Teutsch, a friend and longtime colleague, wrote: "This is in no way a dispute over so-called 'paternity,' however it might have been abusively interpreted in the press. . . . From all evidence, it appears that the event was not seen in the same way on one side or the other, which is not particularly unusual. On the side of Roussel-Uclaf, the people involved do not seem to have been aware of your ideas about eventual compounds of antiprogesterone action, while on your side, it seems that there was a misunderstanding of our activity which brought us to antihormones."

In any collective activity, individuals also act independently; one is not always thinking of what one's colleagues are doing. After the synthesis, all of us made a plan to coordinate biological and clinical study, and we worked as a team.

At Roussel-Uclaf, Teutsch was helped greatly by Alain Bélanger, a Canadian postdoctoral fellow, and Daniel Philibert, a pharmacologist who tested the molecule on animals.

Over the years, the company had synthesized promising steroids which had never been used beyond research. To determine whether RU-486 had practical applications, we had to test its effectiveness on the female cycle. Also, we had to calculate the weakest efficient dosage, prove the constancy of its effect, study how long it remained active, and look at its possible toxicity and long-term effects.

We wanted to design short tests and, to examine the antiprogesterone value, try either to interrupt the menstrual cycle in nonpregnant women or to terminate a pregnancy at its beginning. In principle, we needed to effect only a brief interruption of the women's progesterone flow—this would make for much less expensive testing, and the company was not ready to underwrite long toxicity studies in order to prove RU-486 safe. Checks were favorable. We knew that the metabolism of steroids is fast and that the body eliminates them without leaving any residue. Their effects are reversible; normal activity resumes as soon as they are gone. Over time, my colleagues and I had done a number of experiments on ourselves, including some with compounds made radioactive by tritium or carbon-14. Preclinical tests would be done on two species of animals, of both sexes.

During the summer of 1981, rats were tested at Romainville. Each received 400 mg of RU-486 a day (an enormous quantity considering a rat's weight) with no ill effects. At the same time, laboratories at Huntingdon, England, gave proportionately large amounts to monkeys. By autumn, I began to wonder what was happening with the English monkeys. Then, at a Roussel meeting having nothing to do with RU-486, someone remarked, with a hint of a snicker, "Your compound is dead."

At the highest dose tested, three of the six monkeys showed signs similar to those of serious adrenal insufficiency: fatigue, low blood pressure, a weight loss so serious that after two weeks they were put to sleep to prevent suffering. Adrenal insufficiency symptoms occur when the adrenal glands are destroyed or unable to synthesize corticosteroids, such as cortisol. In the absence of treatment, this is seen in serious forms of Addison's disease.

In this case, as might be expected, the enormous doses of RU-486 had produced a strong antiglucocorticosteroid effect. It was a normal endocrinological reaction. The toxicology report noted that adrenal activity had increased greatly; the cortisol rate was very high and the adrenal glands were enlarged. If you block the effect of glucocorticosteroids with RU-486, the insufficiency of cortisol action brings on a strong pituitary reaction that augments adrenal volume and secretions. In normal circumstances, this adrenal function corrects the lack of hormonal activity in the body. In the case of the monkeys, the huge excess of RU-486 had provoked adrenal reaction, but despite the increase of cortisol, there were signs of adrenal failure.

Thus, the antiglucocorticosteroid activity of the compound was proven, not its toxicity. I insisted on this point, and was able to rescue RU-486 from an early demise.

RU-486 was ready now for tests on women. It was clear that perfecting a new method of interrupting pregnancy would have consequences beyond the normal range of science and medicine. Someone who was competent, but also courageous, would have to take charge of the first clinical tests. No one seemed better suited than my friend Walter Herrmann in Geneva.

Herrmann, above all, is a doctor who cannot neglect his calling; he understands, he treats, he cures. For years, I have sent him those closest to me, and we were bound by our reverence for Raymond Vande Wiele, chairman of obstetrics and gynecology at Columbia University, who had worked with Lieberman. Herrmann, born in Berlin, had studied at Yale and Columbia. His ideas are often ahead of their time. He works with an artist's sensibility and a taskmaster's zeal. I knew he would miss nothing and tell me everything.

Frenchmen later asked me the obvious: Why not in France? One answer was because I wanted to add the weight of the Swiss ethics committee. But for all my admiration and friendship for some specialists in France, I don't think they would have done better.

Herrmann administered RU-486 to eleven women. The dosage was calculated by observing the drug in animals, taking into account the levels of progesterone in women at the start of pregnancy. All went well with the first nine patients: bleeding, expulsion, and a return to the normal cycle, with hardly any cramps and only a little fatigue.

Walter exulted over the telephone. No one had ever heard

of a nontoxic substance, taken orally, that could produce a safe abortion. We had to publish. A first article would announce the clinical results and explain the biological characteristics of RU-486, which were still under wraps. We would discuss eventual applications in reproduction control.

Happily, if one can look at it that way, the next two cases failed as we were editing the text. We might have stopped after nine cases and declared, honestly but inaccurately, that RU-486 was 100 percent effective for abortion. Spontaneous miscarriages, usually provoked by chromosome abnormalities in the embryo, normally are incomplete in one out of five cases, and retained tissue must be removed by curettage. Two failures in eleven patients was not that surprising.

These results, if encouraging, had no statistical validity. They were later confirmed by tests on a larger scale, also with RU-486 alone: 80 percent effectiveness, well-tolerated, corrected adrenal action, with occasional hemorrhage requiring curettage. Herrmann noted that the rate of prostaglandin in the blood went up during the termination of pregnancy. That immediately suggested that using a complementary dose of a prostaglandin derivative could help the process in case of incomplete expulsion. We knew that Marc Bygdeman, Nils Wiquist, and others in Sweden had tested the abortive effects of synthetic prostaglandins.

It was evident that we could induce an abortion. However, we had not shown conclusively that an antiprogesterone and not an antiglucocorticosteroid effect was involved in prenancy interruption. Research on animals would have to suffice. The authorities could hardly expect us to perform experiments on humans. Imagine giving a placebo to a woman seeking to terminate her pregnancy.

The next stage was to improve the rate of success of RU-486. But already we had found a medical alternative to surgical abortion. This was a breakthrough.

At each step of the way, I was only partly aware of what it all meant. Maybe some scientists can foresee all the ramifications of their discoveries, can step back and shout, "Eureka." Not me. The impact of RU-486 came to me progressively, as an international human drama unfolded.

From the beginning, I was after a hazy dream, guided more by instinct than strategy. I learned, little by little, as time went on. Progress came by keeping in contact with people, broadening rather than constricting my focus. Lieberman had taught me that even one person's failure might be the key to someone else's later success. Most people imagine that a scientist declares a fixed, specific goal. I never did center on a single theme. In any case, I'm not ambitious enough to say I want one thing and nothing else. Things have a way of changing their importance in time.

Probably, I reacted as a Frenchman of a certain generation. Until the 1960s, we had no contraception, no legal abortion, just as we hadn't for centuries. We took having a baby very seriously, and pregnancy could be a tremendous problem. The woman decided what to do, and the man's duty was to help. If you were a doctor, you had to decide how to respond.

Abortions were much more common then. Some women had eight, even ten. The method was D and C, as it had been in ancient times. There were two choices. A woman could have a doctor do it clandestinely, which could mean an inordinately high fee and a legal risk. Or if she was poor or without connections, she did it the way women still do in many places. She inserted a stick to provoke a miscarriage and then went to the hospital, where doctors were obliged to repair the damage.

As a young resident, I was shocked by an attitude which seemed to prevail among older doctors. Surgeons would tell their assistants not to bother with anesthesia. "Teach her a lesson she will remember," I heard one of them say.

My first thought was to find a contraceptive that would spare women from abortion. As it turned out, our discovery spanned a broader range. "Contragestion" is an awkward word, but it will make its way. However much anti-abortionist forces seek to draw a line, there is an important middle ground between preventing fertilization and surgically removing a fetus.

RU-486 will allow women to act early on a decision not to pursue a pregnancy. The pill's most dogmatic opponents are men, who often miss this significance. Few women who choose abortion are happy about what they feel they must do. As the embryo develops, an emotional attachment grows. We doctors hear this regularly, in subtle changes of phrase. At first, a woman says she is late. When tests confirm it, she says she is pregnant. Only later, as time goes on, does she say she is expecting a baby.

Pincus, Rock, and Chang gave women a way to prevent conception in the first place. RU-486 lets them act in the following stages. This progression helped me realize what I had been able to contribute. When I received the Albert Lasker Clinical Research Prize in 1989, Chang was there. He was ageless, in his eternal navy blue suit, with his enigmatic smile. He stepped from the crowd to seize my hand. It felt, to me, like a passing of the torch.

Chapter Four

THE
FRENCH
EXPERIENCE

THE SECOND ANNIVERSARY of RU-486's registration came and went in France with hardly a stir. No one
bothered to protest. It worked. Patients liked it and
returned to it. More than one in four abortions were performed
with it, over sixty thousand by the end of 1990, and the percentage was rising. For all the political turmoil, science and medicine
had advanced, and the lives of women were better for it.

Contrary to some early fears, RU-486 did not allow women
to act capriciously. Mifegyne fell under the same French law that
regulated surgical abortion. It was sold only under strict controls,
in authorized family planning center pharmacies, and every box
was accounted for. No black market developed, and doctors did
not try to circumvent established procedures.

RU-486's success was remarkable, not only because doctors
could have been slow to try such a radical new drug but also
because of the brief period in which women may use it in France.
In France, RU-486 is used only up to seven weeks after the last
period.

In British clinical tests, the compound showed the same rate
of effectiveness as in France—96 percent—up to sixty-three days
after the start of the last period. That is two weeks more than the
current limit in France, which is likely to be extended. Many
women hardly have time to make their decision about pregnancy
before the legal French deadline for RU-486.

Anti-abortion sentiment ran high at times. In spasmodic
outbursts, bands of activists burst into family planning centers
and smashed equipment in protest to what they called murder.

The commandos called themselves "Operation Sauvetage," a translation of Operation Rescue in America.

To some, I remained a monster of particular import. One medical colleague liked to call me an "amalgam of Joseph Stalin and Adolf Hitler." Extrapolating from my optimistic forecasts of how RU-486 could be used by a billion women in the Third World, he accused me of plotting the death of several billion young human beings. One small group of extreme rightists took out an advertisement falsely accusing the French Anti-Cancer League of funding our abortion research. It denounced "Etienne Blum, alias Baulieu."

Anti-abortion groups sought to have RU-486 banned in the courts. France had just ratified a European charter on children's rights, which said: "Every child has an inherent right to live." The abortion law of 1975, they argued, violated the charter. French judicial authorities ruled against them.

But active protests remained at the fringe. Doctors with moral reservations concerning abortions simply followed their consciences and referred patients elsewhere. Some physicians who opposed abortion had written Roussel-Uclaf in 1988 to say they would boycott its products. There was no way to know if they did, certainly not from the profit-and-loss statement.

RU-486 caught on fast. There was a run on family planning centers. One of the first patients, a French-American student from Texas, named Sarah, told me about her experience. At twenty-three, with no job or clear idea of how to shape her life, the last thing Sarah needed was a child. She had stopped the contraceptive pill because of side effects, but then she met a man who made her wish she had not. At the end of the month, she began a long wait. Hoping against hope for a simple late period, she waited weeks. Finally, she went to a gynecologist, who confirmed her fears.

"I had read about RU-486 and wanted to try it," Sarah said. "The doctor would not do any abortions for moral reasons, but she gave me a list of clinics. I was right on the borderline, and all of the places had long waiting lists. By the time they could get to me, it would be too late. I called back my doctor, who sent me to a man she knew. He saw how desperate I was and told me to come in the next day."

Sarah waited out the seven-day "period of reflection" legally required for all abortions, took the pills, and returned for the prostaglandin injection.

"When I came in at nine o'clock, they put me in a room and gave me a shot," she said. "They told me I'd feel pain in an hour and would start bleeding in two hours. They were right. The pain was like menstrual cramps, twenty times over, but it passed. At two o'clock, they said I could go home. By then I felt fine, physically and mentally. It wasn't like being in a hospital. No gown or anything. It was just in case something happened, but nothing did. It felt more like a hotel. I just sat around and watched television: 'Who's the Boss?' dubbed in French."

Sarah said her bleeding continued for three days, more than during a period, and then it was just a little for the next twelve. Unlike nearly all Frenchwomen, she was not covered by the state medical plan which pays 80 percent of the bill. The RU-486 and medical charges, including a last checkup two weeks later, cost her about what a surgical abortion would have cost.

Soon after Sarah's experience, we began decreasing the dose of prostaglandin, and we sought new procedures of administering it to reduce cramps.

No one took the pill home. Roussel-Uclaf wanted to prevent any risk of a black market in RU-486, and French authorities shared the company's concerns. Doctors worried about what I call the "cousin effect." A woman might receive the compound under controlled circumstances but, if she were allowed to take it home for whatever reason, she might change her mind, not take the compound, and leave it in her medicine cabinet. Some time later, her cousin, pregnant for months, asks her advice, and she remembers the magic pill.

This would be a particular problem with ectopic pregnancies, which develop outside of the uterus, usually in the fallopian tube. If untreated, these can be fatal. Because of sexually transmitted diseases, the incidence of ectopic pregnancy is rising above 5 per 1,000 cases. RU-486 does not stop ectopic pregnancies.

By carefully monitored regulations, only authorized centers are allowed to purchase RU-486. Their pharmacies receive a special register with counterfoils, and supply doctors only the exact amount needed. Before taking the drug, each patient signs a consent form in duplicate. The package label is affixed to the original form and kept with her records. The duplicate stays on file for three years with the pharmacy. There is nothing casual about taking the pill.

Not only curiosity but also eagerness for something new brought a wave of early candidates. When the word went around that we would be testing the product, in the fall of 1982, letters came in fast.

RU-486 was free in its trial stages. After the trials were completed, doctors would not give it up while awaiting government approval, but no price was immediately fixed. Roussel-Uclaf wanted to charge 500 francs (about $80) for one dose of 600 mg to recover its investment within about ten years. The company estimated it had spent 200 million francs, about $35 million, directly on research and development. But how does one calculate all the blind alleys and extra work indirectly related to the product?

The Ministry of Health objected to the 500 francs; the price could be lower if the product was also sold abroad, they said. The French government ends up paying most pharmacy bills, via social security, and it watches pricing carefully. The ministry suggested 90 to 100 francs, which was just over the cost of manufacture. Roussel-Uclaf refused, pointing out that it could not spread its earnings over a wider base. Hoechst forbade export outside of France. After a long, hard dialogue, a compromise was reached at the beginning of 1990; the price was fixed at 263 francs.

By the end of 1990, almost 600 of the 850 French centers licensed to perform abortions had used RU-486. One of the first to sign up, at Broussais Hospital in Paris, is run by a no-nonsense gynecologist who fights hard for women's rights, Dr. Elisabeth Aubény. Her clinic is homey, with plants and big blue chairs, but its walls reflect the tone. Posters announce women's self-help sessions and support groups, and a phone number for battered wives. Dr. Aubény's brisk but friendly tone keeps patients at ease and staff members on alert.

The clinic performed trials with RU-486 from 1984 to 1988, before Mifegyne was put on the market. The idea fit in with Dr. Aubény's philosophy that women should be responsible for their own bodies. RU-486 not only reduced the complications of surgical abortion, but also allowed patients to take part in the process.

Dr. Aubény is careful to advise patients what RU-486 is not. She does not sugarcoat the pill. It takes more time than surgery, she warns, and it takes a commitment.

"We tell the women that they have to take themselves in hand," she explains. "If they don't want to know anything or see anything, this is not the right method for them. Most women say that they want to avoid surgery, to have an abortion without aggression, as with aspiration. They tell us they want to take charge of themselves, to direct their own abortion. They start the process, watch for signs of an abortion at home or at the clinic, and often they are the ones who decide when it is over. They cannot hide it from themselves because they see the expulsion. This method demands a great deal of responsibility, but women prefer it. There are a few, and this is quite rare, who say that the method is too long, too complicated, and they choose another method."

A printed form lays out the procedure. On the first visit, heart patients, heavy smokers, and asthmatics are screened out because of possible prostaglandin complications. If there are no contraindications, and if it is less than forty-two days from the beginning of her last period, the woman qualifies for RU-486. She must then wait the required seven days of reflection.

On a second visit, she takes three pills of RU-486 in the doctor's presence and goes home with a third appointment for thirty-six to forty-eight hours later. Bleeding sometimes starts before then. Back at the clinic, she is given prostaglandin, by injection or vaginal suppository, and rests for about four hours.

Expulsion occurs during this time, in most cases, or in the next twenty-four hours. Before leaving the center, she is prescribed an oral contraceptive to take for the next month. A final visit fifteen to nineteen days later confirms that no fetal tissue is left behind.

"The choice is up to the woman, and at least 80 percent of women who have tried both methods prefer the pill," Aubény said. "When they are undecided, we guide them toward RU-486, especially if it is early, because we think there is less chance of a problem. Before six weeks, there are too many complications with aspiration."

Although the method is usually spread over a longer period than surgical abortion, there is only one extra visit. Since many surgical patients in France spend a night in the hospital, the actual time involved can be less with RU-486, and costs are lower. There is less chance of tissue remaining with RU-486 than with surgery.

Christiane Der Andreassian, a tall, blond mother of two boys, is a nurse at the clinic and a source of its good-natured atmosphere. Her manner relaxes patients, and she spends hours answering questions.

"The questions that foreigners ask—Americans, for instance—are identical with those asked by the French," she said. "It is always the same problems, women's problems. Those who come here early enough for the RU usually are a certain type. They listen fairly well to their bodies. The other category who come here have no real accord with their bodies and come in much later. It takes them almost two missed cycles to realize, 'Aha, there is something wrong here.' "

Christiane is a practicing Catholic; like a lot of French people, her feelings are mixed. She told her eight-year-old son not to tell the teachers at his private school that she works at the clinic. Relating this to me, she recalled:

"He thought for a bit and then said to me, 'You know, *maman*, there are mothers and fathers who don't spend time with their children, and some of them don't really love their children, and it probably would be better if they had not had those children, if they don't love them.' For me, it's very important that he understands this.

"I began working in an emergency room in 1967, before abortions were legal. We had women come in who had induced their own abortions or who had had clandestine abortions. They had infections or had lost a great deal of blood, and often there was nothing we could do. Many of them died. Those experiences convinced me that we needed a safe and humane way for women to choose to terminate their pregnancy. I would never say that the RU is an easy thing to do, but instead of just going through the motions, this method makes you stop and reflect."

The clinic gave detailed questionnaires to 130 women, including 13 who had tried other methods earlier. Three did not answer, and 3 others wrote only generally about their experience. All the rest said they chose RU-486 because it seemed more natural and avoided surgery. Of those, 116 pronounced themselves satisfied; 8 said the process was too long, with too much responsibility.

A sampling of patients at the clinic suggests a wide range of reaction.

Danielle, a thirty-year-old accountant in a modeling agency, laughed easily about her experience, reflecting a clear idea of what she wanted:

"At the time [February 1990], I had just had a child—he was four months old—and I found out that I was pregnant. I was devastated and overwhelmed. We have another boy, only a year and a half old, and it was out of the question to keep this new pregnancy, financially or physically.

"I was on the pill when this happened, so I suppose mistakes happen. A friend told me about RU, so I called the Broussais center, and they explained the procedure, and I agreed to go through with it. The abortion itself was like a very heavy period. For me, it didn't work right away at the clinic. I went home and suddenly felt I had to pee, and there it was. In between, I was really worried and kept asking myself if this would work and what would I do if it didn't?

"I was amazed at the ease of it all. I hate to say it, but it was

simple. It was much easier than the surgical method, which I
have had before. It was mentally less traumatic than going into a
hospital. The atmosphere at the clinic helps a lot as well. They
are much more at ease, and it seems less stressful. I was very
pleased. It is the answer to a woman's dilemma. I am amazed at
the reaction in the United States to this method. I find it appalling and sad that people would not accept a more sensitive way to
deal with an unwanted pregnancy, one which isn't planned and
can cause problems for the family and the child."

Hélène, who is also thirty, is an accountant, is single, and
lives with her boyfriend. She was ill at ease talking about her
abortion. Tugging repeatedly at her black ski jacket, tucking one
leg under the other, she spoke in a low monotone except when
she asserted, almost violently: "I don't regret it, I had to do
this." Then, more deliberately, she added: "I suffer, and I know
this will always make me suffer, but I do not regret it."

She explained: "I didn't want to have an abortion. I wanted
to keep it, but my boyfriend didn't want it. It is not worthwhile
having a child the father doesn't want. I had heard about RU on
television, and when I needed help, I remembered. I knew right
away I was pregnant, after fifteen days. I felt it in my breasts.
The first time, seven years ago, I didn't feel anything at all, but
this time I was sure. Last time, I had a curettage because the
pregnancy was more advanced, ten weeks. Without anesthesia, I
felt everything that was happening, and it took place on an operating table. I was in pain for a week.

"I didn't know anything about the process except that it
dislodges the egg from the uterus. It produces contractions, like
a miscarriage. And it really hurts. The contractions are strong.
After the prostaglandin I had contractions for two days. But it is
much better than aspiration. The most important thing was to
avoid a hospital stay and surgery.

"It distresses me all the time from the point of view of my
conscience. The first one has always been on my conscience, and
I know this will be as well. But I had to choose, and I chose: it
was the hardest choice of my life. It didn't take me long to
decide because it was what I had to do. But it stays in my mind

because it was a baby. You see, as soon as I felt I was pregnant, it was fabulous. I could tell by all sorts of little things. For instance, with coffee. I love coffee, but one morning when I smelled it I felt like throwing up. I knew it wasn't me, it was someone else. But I had to do it, and I was glad that I was able to choose to do it this way. It was not easier, but more natural, less sterile."

Another thirty-year-old woman, a shoe clerk named Annette, found herself pregnant by a man she met in passing. She had a similar reaction:

"I had already had an abortion, by aspiration, last year. The pill was a lot less difficult. The procedures are basically the same, leading up to it. The social workers often pose the biggest problem. They try to find out why you want an abortion and often they are against it, and they try to make you feel guilty. You feel guilty already, and here's someone else pointing out your failure. They want you to find other ways to solve the problem, but for me there was no other way.

"The pill is much less traumatic, less hard. The clinic here doesn't have the same feeling as the hospital. With aspiration, you are in a bed, under anesthesia. You go into a room and there are all these lights around, and all the people around you. You are lying down watching the people and waiting for it to happen. It is much more traumatizing. It's a lot easier to live through this.

"For the PG [prostaglandin], we were three young women, all sitting in the waiting room. When my contractions started, it hurt a lot, and I wondered if it was normal. But I saw other women were experiencing the same symptoms, and we smiled at each other. I suffered more with the pill than with the aspiration. When you wake up after the aspiration, you feel hardly anything. You suffer a great deal with the pill. It is as though you are having painful cramps. One woman fainted from the pain. You have to live it. Everything we do, we do by ourselves. With the other ways, you are in the hands of the doctor.

"I had never heard of this until I received the results of my pregnancy test. I went to see my doctor and starting crying. I didn't want to go back to the hospital. I couldn't go back on the operating table. It was far too traumatic. So she suggested the pill."

Cost was seldom a factor in a woman's choice of method. In France, few patients pay more than 20 percent of their medical costs. Supplementary expenses like the ultrasonic test are necessary whatever the method, and social security pays in any case. And even without subsidy, costs are comparable. When RU-486 went on the market, a surgical abortion without general anesthesia, and with a hospital stay of less than twelve hours, came to about 850 francs. The treatment with RU-486 and a prostaglandin was in the same range. General anesthesia is more frequently required by women seeking abortion than most people believe. Perhaps because they do not want to face, on the gynecologic table, how vulnerable they may be. Anesthesia requires an additional doctor and expert personnel, increasing the cost significantly.

In most countries, RU-486 will offer potential savings for whoever pays. If it is widely used around the world, the price of the pill will be substantially lower. Surgeons or anesthetists are rarely needed. Clinic visits are brief except for the few hours of observation after taking prostaglandin. Hospital administration costs can be lower. Especially in Third World countries, the use of RU-486 will reduce complications from surgery and anesthesia, which can mean expensive long-term treatment. As methods are perfected to give pills that combine RU-486 with oral prostaglandin, costs can be further reduced, since women will not have to return for an injection.

The cost was one thing. For women who set a value on alleviating traumatic pain, RU-486 seemed a much better deal.

As RU-486 went into distribution, Roussel-Uclaf's clinical coordinator, Louise Silvestre, put together a survey of 2,115 women, laboriously recording every detail to be assembled and compared by computers. Each had a single 600 mg dose of mifepristone followed 36 to 48 hours later by one of two prostaglandins: gemeprost (a 1 mg vaginal suppository) or sulprostone (0.25, 0.375, or 0.5 mg by injection). They stayed in the clinic for 4 hours after taking the prostaglandin.

Overall, the study confirmed earlier results. Ninety-six percent of the women expelled the embryo completely, with no need for any further procedure. Of the failures, 2.1 percent were incomplete expulsions and another 1 percent continued pregnancies, both requiring ordinary surgery. In 0.9 percent of the cases, aspiration was necessary because of excessive bleeding.

At the highest dose of sulprostone, expulsion time averaged 4.5 hours. At the lowest, the mean time was 19.3 hours. With gemeprost, it took 22.7 hours. Uterine bleeding lasted 8.9 days on average. The shortest time was 1 day; the longest was spotting over 35 days. Most of the women had passing abdominal pain from the prostaglandin, but there were few other side effects.

The amount of hemorrhage was no greater than with aspiration. Nothing was learned about any damage to the embryo in a continued pregnancy. A report on the survey in *The New England Journal of Medicine* in March 1990 noted: "We conclude that the administration of mifepristone followed by a small dose of a prostaglandin analogue is an effective and safe method for the early termination of pregnancy."

Later in 1991, Roussel-Uclaf completed a second detailed survey, this time with 16,000 women. The results were virtually the same. That was convincing enough evidence to allay concerns. But we must continue to keep watch carefully. Rare accidents may occur, whether because of individual pathology, or the effects of malnutrition, smoking habits, and stress. All active drugs—indeed all medical interventions—carry a risk, however slight.

Also in 1990, Roussel-Uclaf hired an independent organization to poll doctors at typical centers which used Mifegyne and at others which did not. Two principal conclusions emerged:

"One, the medical method has, in the eyes of doctors (those who prescribe Mifegyne and those who do not), the great advantage of better preserving the gynecological future of their patients." That is, RU-486 spared them the risks of uterine infection or scars, perforation, or cervix dysfunction, not to speak of anesthesia complications.

"The other, the surgical method, has an advantage that might not have been expected: a psychological experience that, in the end, could be less traumatizing for women." In France, many surgical abortions are performed under general anesthesia. Some women report physical or psychic pain, and others do not.

The survey found that the main reason that clinics did not use Mifegyne was because they were too small, with limited administration staff to handle both options. Sixty to seventy percent said they would soon offer RU-486.

I was pleased with the results. After more than a year of comparative use, RU-486 was judged to be safer than surgery. Although doctors like Aubény made a point of emphasizing the commitment required—they did not want women seeking a miracle cure for abortion—the procedure was hardly more time-consuming than surgery. The pain women experienced would be greatly reduced with the use of a different prostaglandin.

All patients had to make an initial visit to ask for an abortion and have an examination. And all of them needed a follow-up visit when it was over. RU-486 required an extra step: returning for prostaglandin. Even that, we felt, would be eliminated after we perfected prostaglandin administration.

For all the good news during 1990, we were worried by two cardiac incidents set off by the prostaglandin. Both women had to be treated for coronary spasms. Each had had earlier histories of heart trouble.

Natural prostaglandins in the body affect all smooth muscles, not only of the myometrium, the muscle of the uterus, but also in the circulatory system and digestive tract. The small dose of synthetic prostaglandin given after RU-486 acts principally within the uterus, which is made sensitive by the antiprogestin. But it also may have an effect elsewhere.

After the incidents, Roussel-Uclaf sent a letter to doctors underscoring the contraindications. Prostaglandins should not be given to women with a cardiovascular risk, including high blood pressure and diabetes, or those with asthma or severe bronchitis. Special care was stipulated for women over thirty-five, particularly smokers.

The letter warned that patients should take prostaglandin while lying down, and blood pressure should be monitored every half hour over the following few hours. Drugs for controlling coronary spasm should be at hand.

These precautions were only for the additional drug. Contraindications for RU-486 itself are chronic adrenal failure, anemia, clotting disorders, long-term steroid or anticoagulant therapies and kidney or liver failure. It also should not be used when there is suspicion of ectopic pregnancy, where an embryo has implanted before reaching the uterus.

The stringent rules were intended to err on the side of caution, and we stepped up our efforts to find a prostaglandin that would be better tolerated.

In 1991, I suggested to Elisabeth Aubény that we begin clinical trials of RU-486 with misoprostol, an orally active prostaglandin already on the market. It is manufactured by Searle of Chicago as Cytotec, and it is for the treatment of stomach ulcers. Ironically, Cytotec shared the front pages of American newspapers along with RU-486 back in 1988 when Roussel-Uclaf sought to suspend the latter. American anti-abortionists failed to block approval for misoprostol even though it has potential as an abortifacient. In fact, particularly in countries where abortion is illegal, women have used misoprostol to induce the start of an abortion, thus obligating doctors to surgically terminate incomplete expulsions.

After clearing the trials with the Broussais Hospital ethics committee and scientific authorities, we bought misoprostol in pharmacies. I decided to inform Roussel-Uclaf and Searle only after we had results to report. Such experimental research with drugs on the market is common practice. But this was delicate ground, and I did not want to mix clinical studies with other concerns.

The results were exciting. Among the first 200 women, 195

had complete expulsion, almost 70 percent within four hours of taking the oral prostaglandin. With the next 75 patients, the success rate was 100 percent. Women reported little pain, and bleeding was no more than with aspiration. By administering prostaglandin orally, we dampened the shock to the system caused by an injection.

Cytotec had amply proven its safety. Four million boxes a year are sold in thirty countries, with sixty pills to a box. We used a single dose that was below that normally taken daily by ulcer patients over the period of several weeks. The manufacturer's recommended dose for gastric treatment is 800 micrograms, taken half in the morning and half at night, for weeks at a time. With RU-486, we gave one dose of 400 micrograms.

The price was an added bonus. Injectable sulprostone costs about 100 francs per dose. Four hundred micrograms of misoprostol cost 4 francs.

More complete trials would be necessary. Although Searle and Roussel-Uclaf each politely declined to associate themselves with our first results (in truth, we had not asked them to), neither closed the door. And within weeks of our publication of results in May's *Comptes Rendus*, the French Ministry of Health wrote to Roussel asking officially that the company test the use of misoprostol with RU-486. The Spanish authorities did the same.

A tragic coincidence added urgency to finding safe oral prostaglandin for use with RU-486. Just as I was finishing the report on the misoprostol-associated regimen for the Academy of Sciences late in March of 1991, André Ulmann telephoned me. A thirty-one-year-old woman in northern France had died of heart failure after an injection of sulprostone following RU-486. She was a chain smoker, and she was terminating her thirteenth pregnancy.

As a result of the incident, Health Ministry officials ordered family planning centers to reduce by half the dose of sulprostone. They banned the treatment for regular smokers and women over thirty-five. Also, they urged that a method be found to administer oral prostaglandin. Misoprostol seemed like an answer.

The death was one too many, but it was the only one among 70,000 women who were given prostaglandin along with RU-486. The outlook had not changed for RU-486 and its potential for the rest of the world. In Britain, the only prostaglandin used is a vaginal suppository, with slower, safer resolution than an injection. The orally active prostaglandin is likely a further improvement.

Sheldon Segal, in an editorial in 1990 accompanying our large-scale survey report in *The New England Journal of Medicine*, had mentioned the company's reluctance to sell RU-486 abroad before it had established itself in France. He wrote, "The new findings . . . provide reassurance on these issues and could presage the availability of the method in countries where comparable conditions of authorized clinical use prevail."

As usual, Sheldon had put his finger on the most sensitive point.

Chapter Five

OUT
INTO THE
WORLD

BY THE END OF 1990, the long-term results in France had left no doubts about the safety and effectiveness of RU-486. Hoechst's most recalcitrant directors, faced with overwhelming evidence of success from further studies, agreed to give the embattled molecule some latitude to make its way in the world. But only on a stringent case-by-case basis.

For all the controversy over the abortion pill, health authorities and family planning groups were clamoring for it in several countries, and many more were interested. It was available only in France, and that was because the government had forced the company's hand. Late in 1990, with leverage from WHO, it was also to be distributed in the largest country in the world.

China had expressed enthusiasm for RU-486 almost as soon as it was announced. The Chinese had already legalized abortion in 1957, and Chinese doctors were among RU-486's first pioneers. I traveled to China three times, beginning in 1983, to talk to specialists about the drug. They saw its possibilities immediately. The Chinese government authorized its use a few days before France approved it.

The Chinese, understandably, were in a hurry. Their 1990 census would show a population of 1.3 billion people. That equals the entire population of the world before World War I. For all its rigor in enforcing population controls, China was falling behind on its goals. In a single generation, the population increase exceeded the government's hopeful projections by 200 million. That's as if an unexpected new nation nearly as populous as the United States had suddenly sprung up in China since 1970.

Within a few weeks of official approval in France, Chinese authorities telexed Roussel-Uclaf to arrange a meeting to discuss distribution. Dr. Qiu Shu Hua, of the State Family Planning Commission, cited favorable results and added: "I request Roussel-Uclaf to consider the best method to supply RU-486 to China." No one in Paris could decide what to do with the telex.

At that moment, protesters were damning us as mass murderers. The archbishop of Paris, Jean-Marie Cardinal Lustiger, condemned the product by name as soon as it was registered. He accused us of experimenting on "little Chinamen." Shortly afterward, religious zealots set fire to the St. Michel Cinema over Scorsese's film on the life of Christ. Conservative Roussel directors were shocked to see the lengths to which fanatics might go.

Claude Evin's declaration that RU-486 was the "moral property of women" had the force of a government decree. But he could only speak for Frenchwomen. As Roussel-Uclaf wavered, word came down from Hoechst in Frankfurt. RU-486 was going nowhere beyond French borders until it proved itself at home.

The order was formal. Along with the Chinese, the Dutch were immediately interested in RU-486. Roussel-Uclaf's affiliate in the Netherlands applied for a license. The Dutch authorities approved it in principle, asking for only routine complementary information before final accord. Suddenly, the affiliate withdrew its application.

The Chinese telex lay in a file unanswered, and soon enough the Beijing government was worried about more immediate matters. Students swarmed onto Tiananmen Square, dispersed eventually by tanks and machine-gun fire. The massacre shocked the world. French relations chilled with China, and the unanswered telex was all but forgotten.

In 1989, I was invited several times to speak in China, where specialists wanted to enlist my support. The time was not right. Hoechst's export ban remained in effect. In 1990, Edouard Sakiz went to China to open a joint-venture chemical plant. To no one's surprise, the subject of RU-486 arose.

Roussel-Uclaf was ready to help, Sakiz said, but that would not be easy. Direct talks would face resistance from Hoechst.

Instead, he suggested informally, why didn't the Chinese take a look at the eight-year-old accord between Roussel-Uclaf and WHO?

Back when the agreement was drafted allowing WHO to distribute RU-486, I had expressed my surprise to Sakiz. Why? I asked. "You never know," he had answered. And here was the perfect application. As a WHO member state and a developing country, China could ask the U.N. agency's help in acquiring RU-486. If Roussel-Uclaf refused, it would risk having to cede rights to another company. Hoechst never objected to the WHO contract and does not object now.

In August 1990, Dr. Huang Baoshan at China's family planning agency wrote to Hiroshi Nakajima, director general of WHO, saying he wanted to buy ten thousand boxes of Mifegyne. The product would be used first in five Beijing hospitals and then in two or three other big cities.

"The purchase of Mifegyne from its French manufacturer Roussel-Uclaf cannot be confirmed without your assistance," Huang wrote. "We request your support and understanding in forwarding this requirement for support to the manufacturer. The Chinese women will be grateful for your intervention in their favor, and your organization can trust the State Family Planning Commission to enforce the good use of this product considered in our country as a humanitarian progress."

This time WHO had to come up with an answer. Unlike his Danish predecessor, Halfdan Mahler, who went on to head the International Planned Parenthood Federation, Nakajima was known to be cool toward RU-486. Even more, American aides had warned him to be careful: any WHO action favoring abortion might endanger the American contribution to WHO which makes up a quarter of its annual budget.

The internal politics were complicated. Nakajima had tried to curb work on RU-486 by WHO's Human Reproduction Unit, the semiautonomous body with private foundation funding. WHO spent no money—and had little say—on the unit's research and clinical tests. But its administration fell under the general WHO budget, and its successes brought credit to WHO.

Nakajima backed off only on the firm counsel of Sune Bergström, chairman of WHO's Scientific and Technical Advisory Group.

Nakajima knew he was on thin ice. In 1991, the U.S. State Department would write to him asking assurances that WHO was not advocating RU-486 or funding any trials on methods of abortion.

But the procedure was respected. Two months after receiving Huang's letter to WHO, Nakajima wrote to Sakiz about the request. After WHO was satisfied that the product would be safely stored and distributed in China, he said, "We hope that your company will supply the product." Nakajima's opening phrase, referring to the "long-standing cooperation between our two organizations," was more than courteous formality. It was a reminder of their formal accord.

Nakajima's letter went on to note: "I look forward to our two organizations being able to arrive at a satisfactory pricing arrangement for the public sector in developing countries in the near future so as to enable the request for supply of this product from the Chinese authorities to be met at a price they can reasonably afford."

Sakiz and sympathetic Roussel executives were pleased to see their breakthrough product strike out beyond French borders, but others grimly accepted the inevitable. If the Chinese wanted ten thousand now, they might soon want ten million. Other Third World countries would follow. For little profit, the executives thought the company was risking ill will or worse from a broad constituency which saw abortion as evil.

Complex factors lay beneath the reluctance to export RU-486, and the reasons in France were different from those in Germany. Roussel-Uclaf is a family-founded French company, true to its tradition. Its conservative good taste emerges from its stone headquarters in the Seventh Arrondissement, just steps from Rodin's old studio and the gold-domed Invalides, built by Louis XIV in 1670 as an old soldiers' home, where Napoleon's body now lies. In the lobby, Gaston Roussel, a veterinarian who built a pharmaceutical empire out of a horse serum business, gazes across at his son Jean-Claude.

The facing portraits illustrate an old France that is changing fast. When Gaston died, his two sons went separate ways. One wanted nothing more to do with pharmaceuticals. The other, Jean-Claude, in spite of his love for a fast, free life, took up the family banner; it was how he saw filial duty. But he could not afford to buy out his brother's equal share. With no other choice, a majority of shares were sold to Hoechst A.G. Later, the French government bought in as well in a partial nationalization. Hoechst's investment and connections have benefited the French company over the years. The conflict over RU-486 was an unusual case.

At Roussel-Uclaf, seventeen thousand executives and employees still see themselves as part of a family. When people resign, others look concerned and wonder what is wrong with them. In this sort of atmosphere, certain things are simply not done.

Though equipped with the most sophisticated technology, in the front ranks of space-age medical science, Roussel-Uclaf was built on ideas and attitudes rooted in another time. Unruly demonstrators in gas masks are not part of the picture. Fears of a boycott are one thing. Worse are fears of a stain on the family name.

Hoechst A.G., on the other hand, is big business. Its annual earnings approach $30 billion, as large as the national budget of some countries. Its directors can play a tough game, but they see no reason to risk consumer reprisals over a dispensable product of questionable taste.

Even more, Hoechst is German big business. Any director over the age of fifty remembers the Third Reich. They grew up with the humiliation of being German, paying the price for what their parents had wrought. For them, the risk of being accused of mass murder is grave, and "holocaust" is not just a buzzword for cynical activists to use in mobilizing public opinion. Hoechst's roots go back to the corporate structure of I.G. Farben, which made poison gas for Hitler. These are origins the directors would prefer to forget.

That aside, demonstrations, boycotts, potential lawsuits, all disrupt the smooth course of avoiding surprises, offending no one, and making money. RU-486 was trouble; it meant disorder. Neither trouble nor disorder is welcome in German boardrooms.

And, more specifically, Hilger, the president, was opposed to abortion under any circumstances. If he could avoid selling an abortion pill, all the better.

All of these factors went into the decision on December 15, 1988, by Roussel-Uclaf's governing committee to keep RU-486 in France except, eventually, under conditions they could not refuse.

Roussel supported trials for purposes other than abortion, and it continued to respect its accords with the Population Council, as well as with WHO. But if RU-486 was to be exported for abortion, the company decided, the importing country would have to satisfy five conditions: (1) Abortion must be legal. (2) It must be accepted widely by "public opinion." (3) A suitable prostaglandin must be available. (4) Distribution must be under tight official control, as with narcotics. (5) Patients must sign a letter agreeing to a surgical abortion if the pill failed. In practice, there was a sixth condition: the company would not sanction exports unless ranking government officials urged them to do it.

These conditions remained in force, but during 1990 the resistance began to fade. China was a major step, but not the only one. Hilger gave Roussel-Uclaf the go-ahead to export RU-486 close to home. To Great Britain.

England had to be next. In 1985, at the first British debate on RU-486 at the CIBA Foundation in London, I was struck by the lucidity and moral concern expressed by doctors, scientists, and theologians. The British looked closely at RU-486, tested it, talked about it, fought about it in heated rallies, and then pressed for the right to use it.

British doctors began exhaustive clinical trials of RU-486 shortly after we published the first papers on it. David Baird, who was spending three years with Pincus when I first visited the Massachusetts center, was among the first to rally around RU-486. He tried the compound with prostaglandin, confirming Bygdeman's results in Sweden. His article in *Lancet*, reporting 95 percent effectiveness, appeared in December 1987, too late for us to include in our application to the French Health Ministry, but soon enough to lend weight to our assertions.

Baird was at the conference in Rio de Janeiro when word first went out that Roussel-Uclaf had stopped RU-486. In his presentation, Baird emphasized the potential of the compound in the Third World. Some risks of misuse were inevitable because of limited medical capacities, he said, but these were negligible compared with present risks from poorly effectuated abortion. Faced with a catastrophic situation, developing countries needed RU-486.

Those of us behind RU-486 knew that Britain was a crucial step. It was a major European neighbor, known for its deliberate and cautious approach in matters of public interest. Even more, it was Anglo-Saxon. Americans felt more comfortable with the British and spoke their language. Frenchmen might do strange things where the body is concerned. But the English? If the pill thrived in Britain, the United States could not be far behind.

If the pill would be legal in Britain, the company's subsidiary there, Roussel Laboratories Ltd., was anxious to get started. G. E. Powderham, Roussel director in London, urged Paris to move fast. Scientific progress was often controversial, he wrote to headquarters, and "there have always been nihilists who would have denied us everything from the steam train to anesthetics." He concluded, "*Courage, mes amis.*"

Roussel's medical directors reported that trials were made without a fuss, despite some objection. Since public opinion was largely indifferent, they said, the company had to choose between disappointing right-to-lifers or women who wanted the pill. It would lose more by abandoning its customers than it would gain by abandoning the product. Image and staff morale would suffer.

But the company's December 15, 1988, decision, which left the Chinese telex unanswered, also froze activities in Britain. No ranking official had demanded it.

As the pill was marketed in France, pressure mounted in

England. Unlike China, Britain was next door. Women made the short hop across the Channel and spread the word among friends. Roussel-Uclaf executives could not avoid the reproachful gaze of the British medical community.

In October 1989, Baird joined other eminent British specialists at a conference on RU-486 organized by the Birth Control Trust. They insisted that the compound should be made available not only in Britain but everywhere. Sir Malcolm Macnaughton, of the University of Glasgow, set a firm tone in a preface to the published proceedings:

"The development of mifepristone is an advance in reproductive medicine of the same magnitude as the development of the hormonal contraceptive pill and is the first effective 'medical' method that can be used for termination of early pregnancy. It means that early pregnancies can now be safely terminated without resort to surgery."

He recalled the furor at the Rio conference and noted the high abortion death rate in the Third World. "The developed countries have a duty to the developing countries to help them with this problem, and it is essential that this new drug be made widely available as soon as possible," he wrote. "The political opposition must be overcome so that women in all countries can have access to this new method of termination."

In his presentation, Baird noted that even when contraception was available, its protection was never complete. "I believe that abortion is needed as a backup where contraception fails," he said. "Furthermore, as some 75 percent of countries have some form of legal abortion, it is the responsibility of individuals and governments to ensure that the best medical technology is available to women in those countries."

Madeleine Colvin, legal officer for the National Council for Civil Liberties, explained not only why RU-486 would be legal under Britain's Abortion Act of 1967 but also how far the government or a manufacturer could go "to withhold a proven drug because of pressures exerted upon them by opponents." If a company did not apply for a license, the government could grant the British patent to someone else. And if the government was unwilling to do that, another applicant could sue for the patent after three years.

Allan Templeton, head of obstetrics and gynecology at the University of Aberdeen, reported on three types of clinical trials. First, RU-486 with prostaglandin was up to 96 percent effective in pregnancies of up to nine weeks, which was two weeks longer than the current French limit. Second, it was useful as a cervical primer for women who preferred vacuum aspiration. And third, it significantly reduced side effects and pain when used with prostaglandins for therapeutic abortions in the second trimester. To this last point, he added: "Second-trimester abortion is an unpleasant procedure [and] anything that can lessen its distress is to be welcomed."

Later, Templeton and his colleagues demonstrated another advantage of RU-486 over curettage. Surgical abortion carries the risk that blood from the fetus may mix with the mother's blood, possibly causing Rh-factor problems in a subsequent pregnancy. RU-486 substantially reduces this risk.

In some circles, a paper entitled "The Potential Effects on National Health Service Resources" caught the most attention. Ian MacKenzie, a consultant to the John Radcliffe Maternity Hospital at Oxford, reported on a detailed study of comparative costs to Britain's socialized medical system.

He calculated that a 600-mg dose of RU-486 would cost about 25 pounds (about $48). Adding a prostaglandin and a hospital stay of four to six hours, treatment would come to 75 pounds per patient. Surgical abortions, which require general anesthesia, cost 180 pounds for the day cases, which amount to half of the total. But the other patients spend one or two nights in the hospital, bringing the average cost to 270 pounds.

Basing his figures on 79,000 abortions a year, and factoring in other variables, MacKenzie estimated that RU-486 could save the National Health Service between 10 and 15 million pounds a year, "with an anticipated reduction in patient morbidity, an added advantage."

At the Birth Control Trust Conference, Dilys Cossey, chairwoman of Britain's Family Planning Association, pointed out that any change toward making women more independent has always been resisted. The classic British case is the use of anesthesia in childbirth, which was not accepted until Queen Victoria used it: "we need to find a similar personality today to give RU-486 the endorsement it deserves."

Doctors seconded the Birth Control Trust's position favoring RU-486. In the *British Medical Journal*, John Guillebaud made a convincing case for the pill, not only for early abortions but also to ease more difficult abortions later on. He cited a quotation from Baird: "The valid point for discussion is whether it is ethical to carry out therapeutic abortion under any circumstance. While it is legal to carry out therapeutic abortion, surely it is incumbent on medical scientists to develop safe and effective means which will preserve the health of women."

A safe and effective means had been found, he said, but if it was not legally available, it would be driven underground. British women would use it anyway, but with less safety and effectiveness.

Guillebaud reported that the 1989 meeting of the International Planned Parenthood Federation, in Ottawa, had deplored delays in making RU-486 available to women. "So, I am sure, will most readers of the *BMJ*," he concluded.

There were protests, and a threatened boycott. More than anything else, they showed how a noisy minority can unnerve a pharmaceutical company but do little once a controversial but safe drug is on the market by popular demand and physicians' support.

One anti-abortion organization, Campaign for the Complete Welfare of the Woman and Child, warned: "The abortion pill RU-486 goes one step further; it makes the 'solution' appear even simpler, killing an unborn baby becomes almost wholesome." The group circulated a form for people to give to their doctors, asking that no Roussel product be prescribed for them— unless, the form added, their health depended upon it.

The process of bringing out a new drug is long and costly, with complex patents, and the consumer's choice is not always wide. Companies tend to specialize, and doctors pick drugs for their efficacy rather than their brand name. In reality, a useful, reliable drug is never vulnerable to a long-term boycott.

The exposure is greater for multinational conglomerates that produce a range of products. Consumers might boycott mattress fibers to protest a pill. But other factors apply. If medical science needs the pill, and a large public wants it, a responsible company can withstand what amounts to terror tactics.

Hoechst's shift in attitude came a month after the Birth Control Trust conference in 1989. I don't know why. I only knew that Hilger, a widower, had remarried. In November, he and Sakiz dined together. Afterward, Sakiz called me in a joyful mood. No one could say anything yet, but RU-486 would be crossing the Channel.

In March 1990, Roussel-Uclaf officials made a visit to Frankfurt for strategic planning. One agenda item was applying for a license to sell RU-486 in Britain. Fine, said Hoechst, take the responsibility.

There was still the informal sixth condition. The company wanted a senior government official to invite an application. Soon afterward, Health Minister Kenneth Clarke rose in the House of Commons and declared his firm support for the French pill, which, he said, would allow British women the freedom of choice. No one could be more specific than that. In November 1990, Roussel Laboratories applied for licensing. Since clinical trials had already been completed, the approval process was not expected to take long. Approval came on July 1, 1991.

The British decision was likely to have an impact on Ireland, the last country in Western Europe with a harsh anti-abortion law. Each year, more than 5,000 Irish women travel to neighboring Britain to terminate pregnancies. Dr. Walter Prendiville, a young Dublin professor, has asked Roussel-Uclaf about using RU-486 to treat incomplete abortions, whether spontaneous or illegally induced. This purely medical use was not expected to raise objections, either from physicians or from Mrs. Mary Robinson, the newly elected President.

The next logical place was Scandinavia. RU-486 owed much to Bergström and Bygdeman, who had pioneered work in prostaglandins. Sweden had an intelligent, humane attitude toward family planning. It was the world leader in fertility control, and yet its demographic curve is rising, and has been doing so for several years—a remarkable case in Europe. This disproves the myth that easily available contraception and abortion services tend to reduce populations. RU-486 should be among Scandinavian women's choices.

The Nordic countries fell under the responsibility of Roussel Laboratories in Britain, and Powderham helped set up trials with Yves Sanson, the expert president of Roussel Nordiska A.B. Bygdeman lent his enthusiasm, trying out an extremely active new prostaglandin, meteneprost. The Swedish media response was favorable, and no one raised a voice against RU-486. But, as elsewhere, export was put on hold.

On August 21, 1990, after a meeting of the Professors of Obstetrics and Gynecology in Scandinavia, Bygdeman and thirteen other noted specialists wrote to Roussel-Uclaf: "The unwillingness of your company to provide mifepristone for scientific studies and to market the compound in Scandinavia is unacceptable."

Soon afterward, the company relented. Its policy was still one step at a time. Britain would have to go first, but Sweden would follow. Other Scandinavian countries would likely be next.

With the first export barriers broken, it seemed only a matter of time before a critical mass would build, carrying RU-486 into the European markets and beyond. All of Europe had legalized abortion. Besides Ireland, the last holdout was Belgium, where a Catholic king remained adamant. In April 1990, King Baudouin abdicated his throne for a single day so that the parliament could pass an abortion law he would not have to oppose.

But it would be an uphill struggle for RU-486. In many countries, the company dragged its heels. An application was still frozen in the Netherlands, though it was all but approved in 1988. The open-minded Dutch approach to individual choice, and the government's commitment to the latest in medical advances, virtually guaranteed an enthusiastic reception. But the open minds in Holland worried the more staid minds in France.

Few dared to say it aloud, but some Roussel executives

were uneasy about sending their disputed pill to Amsterdam. Unfocused fears of a permissive drug culture in that city loomed in their imagination. They saw the bogey of a black market. If confronted on these views, Roussel executives might hedge. The Netherlands was hardly a lawless, disorganized state. But deep down there was a sensitivity to criticism.

In Latin countries, mostly Catholic, warm public reaction hailed the first trials of RU-486. But local directors of Roussel-Uclaf sometimes shied away. Unfairly, they argued that distribution could not be adequately controlled, and did not understand how much women now play a part in these changing societies.

Officials acknowledge 80,000 abortions in Spain and Portugal each year—the actual figure may be higher than 400,000—and they are showing interest in RU-486. In April 1991, Ignacio Lobato of the Spanish Health Ministry sent an insistent letter to the Roussel subsidiary asking for trials with RU-486 and misoprostol as a first step toward possible wide distribution. This was a remarkable move, a significant show of respect for women's rights in a country that had to reimplant democracy.

Bitter controversy over the pill broke out in Italy, where sectors of a modernizing society brought science in conflict with politics. A broad range of doctors, officials, and women's organizations demanded that RU-486 be imported. But they ran into a wall of resistance from traditional elements. The Vatican, needless to say, had a major impact.

Italy has one of the most liberal abortion laws in Europe. In 1981, a referendum confirmed the 1978 law that legalized abortion, with a 70 percent majority in favor of abortion. Catholics and men voted heavily in favor. Yet the issue is still caught up in complexities.

As in France and Britain, most surgical abortions must be performed under general anesthesia. This means a woman requires two doctors—a gynecologist and an anesthetist—willing to perform an abortion. Elsewhere, this is seldom difficult. In Italy, however, the Vatican exerts pressure on doctors to decline on the grounds of conscience. Especially in small towns and rural areas, women find it hard to get two doctors for an abortion.

Although there is significant official backing for the pill, the Italian government is invariably balanced on a shaky coalition. Roussel-Uclaf would like a clear positive signal from authorities who can dampen controversy. But no single party can muster enough support to give it, even within the Health Ministry itself.

One of two undersecretaries of health, Elena Marinucci, campaigned vigorously for RU-486, arguing that many Italian women suffered needlessly because of anti-abortion doctors who complicated the system on the strength of the conscience clause. She was a Socialist. The other undersecretary of health, a Christian Democrat, was dead set against RU-486.

"Italy is not like England, where Kenneth Clarke can get up in Parliament and ask for the pill," Marinucci told me once. "Most women want it here, but our politics don't work that way."

The issue rages periodically in the papers, and leading figures wade into the debate. Rita Levi-Montalcini, among the world's most remarkable women and a Nobel laureate in medicine, took up the cause. Applying her charm, force of personality, and the wisdom of eighty years, she stands up to subtle reproaches from the Vatican, which had named her to the Pontifical Academy of Sciences.

In 1990, the prestigious women's organization Club delle Donne made its position clear. They awarded me the first Minerva Prize ever given to a foreigner.

The situation in Italy is complex. Mid-1991 Roussel was to commercialize an antibiotic with an Italian drug company. Representatives of that company were told that an official of the Vatican, influential on the committee delivering registration for drugs, asked for a public declaration by Roussel stating that they would not introduce RU-486 in Italy. Roussel had to do it.

In German-speaking Europe, the distribution of RU-486 is even more up to Hoechst than elsewhere. In Austria, the Ministry of Health officially and strongly asked for trials. Hoechst flatly refused. Abortion is severely restricted in what used to be West Germany.

The law dates back to the 1851 Prussian code. Under Paragraph 218 of the German Reich Penal Code of 1871, a woman guilty of abortion could be imprisoned for five years. The practitioner was liable to a life sentence. Sentences were eased, but Hitler stiffened them again; I learned from Dr. Henry David that abortion was allowed only for Jews! Under today's Paragraph 218, both doctor and patient can be jailed if an abortion is not sanctioned by two specialists as socially and medically necessary. Especially in Bavaria, where the Catholic Church is strong, permission for an abortion is difficult to get.

Before reunification, West German women had the option of "abortion tourism." They could travel to Holland or they could go to East Germany, where abortion was available on demand at state-subsidized rates. With the merger, Chancellor Helmut Kohl's Christian Democratic Party had a problem. Imposing West Germany's law would alienate East Germans. Relaxing it for the whole country would anger the right wing and lose votes among a broad range of fundamentalists.

In mid-1990, Kohl resolved the problem by putting it off for two years. Until then, in the five former East German states, abortions would be legal. And as demanded by the Social Democrats in order to reach a necessary three-quarters majority, no West German woman can be prosecuted for traveling east to have an abortion. Eventually, a new Bundestag will have to write a different law.

The Bundestag president, Rita Süssmuth, a Christian Democrat and a former health minister, argues for a "middle way" which would oblige a woman to visit a counseling center before going ahead with an abortion. But Bavarian hard-liners reject this compromise position.

German women living near Holland have routinely crossed the border for treatment. In early 1991, the magazine Der Spiegel reported that German police stopped a woman suspected of having had an abortion in Holland. She was forced to undergo a medical examination. Interior Ministry officials confirmed there had been two other such cases in recent years. This kind of harassment, said Housing Minister Irmgard Adam-Schwaetzer, was a throwback to the Middle Ages.

Medical opinion on RU-486 was divided from the start. In

1985, Dr. Michael Popovec, of the German physicians' association, decried the pill as dangerous. Even if it proved to be safe clinically, he said, he was against it. "I think mostly of the dangers that such a product would have on the dignity of human nature," he said. On the other hand, Dr. Horst Spielman, a ranking federal health official, praised RU-486 as a necessary alternative to surgical abortion.

As elsewhere, sentiment is growing for the pill. Against this current, Hoechst has stood firm, not only in Germany but also in Austria. In 1990, Hoechst and Roussel-Uclaf turned down an official request for an initial trial of one hundred abortions by the Austrian Ministry of Health.

With the integration of Europe after 1992, however, the situation is likely to change. After the examples of France, Britain, and Sweden, it will be hard to deprive German women of RU-486. Things will move quickly.

As Hoechst resisted bringing its pill to Germany, a major competitor, Schering in Berlin, waited quietly in the wings. Although Roussel-Uclaf was first with its antiprogestin, Schering has developed active analogues. Several might even slip by Roussel-Uclaf's patent, despite being based on the same chemical formula.

After successful abortion tests with animals, Schering took a low profile. Its researchers had to focus on breast cancer research, and they announced that their product was more effective than RU-486 in treating tumors. Roussel-Uclaf held the edge, even in breast cancer research, because its compound was already widely in clinical use, and therefore known as a safe drug.

Frenchmen and Germans understand a classic strategy of bicycle racing. A strong racer may choose to hang back in second place for much of the race until he finds the moment to spurt ahead and take the lead. Schering has yet to take its antiprogestins to clinical trials. No one, however, is counting it out of the race.

The Soviet Union has shown interest in RU-486. They need it badly. Abortion was legalized after the October Revolution, a reaction to strict controls imposed by the czars. Except for restrictions under Stalin, later repealed, the law has been liberal ever since. In the absence of contraceptive methods, abortion is the major means of birth control. It is very cheap and permitted up to the twelfth week of pregnancy. But like so many things in the Soviet Union, it is extremely hard to get.

Official figures estimate abortions at 7 to 8 million a year. This already surpasses the number of births, and is four times the average abortion-to-birth rate in developed Western countries. In fact, more than another 10 million illegal abortions go unreported, performed in back-street apartments or hovels in the countryside. Soviet hospitals cannot meet the demand.

Archil Khomassoridze, director of the Zhordania Institute for Human Reproduction in Tbilisi, Georgia, worries that the situation is growing from crisis to catastrophe. In 1990, he organized a WHO-sponsored conference entitled "From Abortion to Contraception," to explore ways of relieving the pressure. At the meeting, I was peppered with questions about RU-486.

Early in 1991, scientific colleagues and authorities reported that there was general agreement to bring RU-486 to the Soviet Union. Proposals were made either to buy it in quantity or to seek to manufacture it under license.

Later on, the Soviet first vice-minister of health A. A. Baronov asked Roussel-Uclaf to help set up abortion trials. But the request awaited action in Paris.

Elsewhere in eastern Europe, the breakdown of the Communist system has created a unique situation: in all countries but Romania, contraception and abortion were legal and governmentally subsidized. In rejecting Communism, however, these countries, will tend to reevaluate all social practices, including those that may have been favorable to women.

In Poland, the situation is extreme because of the role of the Catholic Church both in undermining the socialist regime and in trying to rule the country. Two-thirds of the population want to maintain strict separation between church and state. Before the Pope's visit in early June 1991, however, the Parliament discussed a new law, a "gift" to the Pontifical Authority. The law would have abolished the ruling established in 1956, and women or doctors involved in abortion would have been punishable by two years of jail. Ironically, it was thanks to the ex-Communist members of the Parliament that the proposal was turned down. But another law was to be prepared and submitted, one certainly less liberal than the present one.

Even in its present state, the Polish situation is a disaster. Abortion is legal, but of the 600,000 abortions a year, 500,000 are performed illegally—often unsafely and always expensively. The 1956 law had permitted abortion, but required the recommendations of two physicians and a psychologist. How can a woman be expected to find three individuals who are not influenced by the Church's position? Especially in the smaller towns or in the countryside? Pharmacists now work under a liberal regime and can sell contraceptives. They face severe threats from religious zealots. The risk of unwanted pregnancy has never been so high, and Polish women suffer.

Traveling in Poland for a scientific meeting, I recently met Wladyslaw Sidorowicz, a psychiatrist and Minister of Health. I suggested to him that Poland perform trials with RU-486 and misoprostol. Several endocrinologists and gynecologists there have relayed their good will, and the local director of Roussel-Uclaf only awaits governmental approval.

Hungarians, with a long tradition in neurobiology and sophisticated gynecology, were quick to understand the promise of RU-486, following in the footsteps of Arpad Csapo, who did pioneer research in the role of progesterone in human pregnancy. The first WHO publication on RU-486 was signed by Lajos Kovacs. But the newly democratized country is governed by a coalition, and, Kovacs observed, the Health Ministry has not yet defined its position.

In Yugoslavia, partisans of RU-486 have also not been able to spur action among government authorities preoccupied with so many urgent problems. Dr. Lidija Andolsek was the most eloquent voice to argue within WHO for the drug's potential in helping the Third World, but she could not raise the issue as a priority in her country.

Elsewhere in the world, bureaucratic difficulties along with varying degrees of moral, social, or religious resistance, suggest an open future for RU-486. Currents in a number of countries in time will swell to a tide that cannot be stopped. Meanwhile, a single well-placed national authority who opposes the product, or who fails to act because of simple inertia, can be enough to stop any proposal.

This seems to be the case in India which, like China, was an early proponent of RU-486. In 1983, Prime Minister Indira Gandhi told me she planned to take steps to introduce the pill. Since then, authorities have expressed official interest. But progress through the bureaucracy has been difficult.

In neighboring Bangladesh, however, authorities are actively discussing the use of RU-486 for menstrual regulation. The Moslem nation limits abortion, but it already offers women vacuum aspiration at the earliest stages of pregnancy. The Ford Foundation helped the Bangladesh Association for Prevention of Septic Abortion (BAPSA) to organize an international conference on introducing RU-486 in Bangladesh; it was postponed during the Gulf War but was rescheduled for October 1991.

The huge Moslem nation of Indonesia is in a position similar to Bangladesh's. Menstrual regulation is tolerated, though not legal, and specialists have asked about RU-486.

Other Islamic countries are divided on the pill. Doctors in Algeria and Tunisia want to introduce RU-486 for early use, as in Bangladesh. Despite some official backing, they face opposition from religious fundamentalists.

In most of Latin America, the Catholic Church bars the way. Abortion, if outlawed, is usually tolerated in Latin American countries. In Brazil, there are more than four million abortions a year, all of them illegal, and the health consequences are catastrophic. But a method as controversial as RU-486 will require political champions to storm the barriers.

Beyond Europe, the most promising frontiers are the other industrialized nations. Japan is an obvious market, and there is already serious interest. In Japan, as in the Soviet Union, birth control depends mostly on condoms and abortion. But the setting is vastly different, and so are the reasons.

Japan's postwar Eugenic Protection Law affords doctors broad leeway in performing abortions. Eugenics seeks to preserve the best qualities inherent in a race, and the Japanese consider it important to control their numbers. In the mid-1950s, there were a million abortions a year. Now the official annual total is about 500,000, but to reach the real figures, I am told, one must multiply that by two or three.

Over the years, the surgeons who performed abortions gained power over the broader field of fertility control in Japan. For their own purposes, they resisted the contraceptive methods that had taken hold in the rest of the world. Only in the past few years have oral contraceptives made a timid entry into Japan. Clearly, financial interests are at stake. An increasing number of Japanese women want RU-486, but the decision is up to their doctors.

When I speak in Japan, I make the point that RU-486 is given under medical supervision. There is no reason it should not be administered by gynecologists, as it is in France, leaving abortion in the same hands as it is now. As a result, doctors are starting to show interest, and RU-486 could have a brighter future in Japan than oral contraceptives.

Sometimes, unexpected obstacles beyond medicine stand between women and the freedom to shape their own lives. This was made clear to me during a tumultuous trip I made to Australia in 1990. Though a country of 17 million inhabitants, Australia has produced or attracted some great scientists in the field of reproduction. Family planning groups and medical colleagues invited me to speak there, and the controversy began even before I left Paris.

A lobbying movement seemed to be afoot in Australia to bring in RU-486. Australia's Socialist government is in favor of the pill. The country's strong advocates have roots in history. In 1937, five thousand Australians filed past the grave of Dr. Albert Bretherton, a local hero who arranged abortions for the poor, paid for by the rich. Jo Wainer, who follows her husband's path in directing the Abortion Providers Federation of Australia, wrote that "for the first time, it really will be possible [for women to be] just a little bit pregnant," and she wants to make use of the Australian Planned Parenthood slogan "if you are late, come early."

The day before my flight to Perth, I learned that the health minister of Western Australia, Keith Wilson, had banned my talk at the King Edward Memorial Hospital for Women. A former Protestant clergyman, he did not accept abortion.

He backed down in the face of protests. Major women's organizations, the Australian Medical Association, and opposition politicians denounced the move as "censorship."

In Canberra, anti-abortion demonstrators gathered outside the National Press Club, but the audience I addressed inside was enthusiastic.

A majority of government ministers had privately declared themselves in favor of RU-486, but none seemed prepared to make the sort of clear statement which Kenneth Clarke delivered to the House of Commons. Without a strong push from the manufacturer, resistance by small but vociferous groups made it unlikely that the pill would be approved in Australia before use in England, a Commonwealth partner which often influences Australia.

I was also saddened to see a curious alliance between some feminist organizations and anti-abortion groups of the extreme right. These feminists argued that as women they had no control over certain methods, such as hormonal contraception and intra-uterine devices, and they rejected them.

Some of these groups recruited doctors to denounce RU-486 from a position of authority, although none had had any experience with it. It was as if I, as a biochemist, had attacked methods of neurosurgery.

Australia was a specific case. But I am always surprised at the obstacles that arise in countries with no legal or cultural reason to resist such a significant advance in medicine. Is it that politicians, mostly men, are so insensitive to their women constituents? Is it that women cannot yet make their voices heard? Or is it a lingering reluctance to confront abortion, a word and deed which no one really likes?

Years after developing RU-486, it still bothers me to be identified as "the" man behind the abortion pill. Not only have several people contributed to its design, I would also like it to be clear that I do research in other fields. And yet the pill represents a great step for medical science: not only a safe backup to contraception but also a way to eliminate classic invasive abortion.

Signs are encouraging that exports of RU-486 will reach a threshold, spreading with increasing ease to different parts of the globe, including North America. In Canada, after Parliament threw out restrictive abortion legislation, the law of the land is a Supreme Court decision that leaves the way clear. There is fresh, widespread interest there among official circles.

But whether RU-486 will fulfill its true promise depends on the main question left hanging: When, and under what conditions, will it enter the United States?

Chapter Six

THE PILL
IN AMERICA

OTHERS DID IT a bit more elegantly, but the *New York Post* captured the American mood in late September 1989: "Furor Over Award for Abort-Pill Doc, Pro Lifers Rip 'Human Pesticide.' " For all its success in France and its promise elsewhere, RU-486 was not yet available in the United States. It was kept out, not by American authorities, but because Roussel-Uclaf, under pressure from Hoechst, sought no license. There was just too much heat.

As one American reporter observed, a principal condition for exporting RU-486—a favorable public and political climate—was French understatement. It meant: no controversy. Roussel-Uclaf directors hoped initially that protests would subside. Now, the proponents of RU-486 in the company are counting instead on reason. And there is cause for optimism.

The uproar in 1989 erupted when I received the Lasker Prize, America's most prestigious medical award. In the *Post*, Gretchen Berger of the National Organization for Women (NOW) exulted, "It's fabulous. This will save women's lives." She predicted the pill's approval after a "down and dirty fight."

The article went on to suggest how dirty the fight might be. It quoted the ubiquitous John Willke of the National Right to Life Committee, who renewed his threat to boycott Hoechst if American women were allowed access to RU-486. Mark Lucas of Operation Rescue was quoted as saying: "Awarding a man who created a human pesticide is despicable."

In accepting the Lasker award, I stressed the point that RU-486 gives women a choice: "Choice is freedom. Science cannot and must not dictate our beliefs. But science can provide choices." And I hoped that American women would soon have the freedom to choose.

I believed from the beginning that RU-486's eventual destiny would be shaped in the United States. The need for it is overwhelming. Half of the 6 million pregnancies a year are unintended. Each year, 1.6 million abortions are reported, a third of them among women under twenty.

America has the highest rate of teenage pregnancy in the developed world, four times as many per capita as the Netherlands. It is distressing to think of so many girls entering womanhood in this way, restrained by stirrups on a clinic operating table.

A huge domestic need is one thing. But even more, much of the world looks to America to lead the way. The first-generation pill was developed in the United States, in the face of virulent hostility. The inspiration that pushed me toward the second-generation pill came largely from American energy. The United States is the leader in advanced research, the main source of development funds, and the heart of worldwide networks which can allow RU-486 to help women everywhere.

In the United States, however, abortion stirs conflict with a force not seen since the Vietnam War, nearly a generation ago. Nothing can be more elemental than the issues of life and death, or a woman's rights in regard to what happens in her own womb.

I have always felt that RU-486 would come to America once enough people understood what it was. Confusion surrounded the pill from its first appearance, as much from disinformation as misinformation. At its most basic level, the dispute was never about science.

On the day RU-486 was licensed in France, Food and Drug Administration specialists came to hear me speak at the National Institutes of Health in Bethesda, Maryland. They wanted to know more. We prepared a background dossier so that they would be prepared when Roussel-Uclaf applied for licensing in the United States. Since then, FDA scientists have followed our progress. Privately, they make it clear: from a technical standpoint, an application for RU-486 almost certainly would be approved.

In a free-ranging democracy like the United States, nothing is immune to politics. Legislators with a point of view to push may not always be convinced by facts.

Early in 1986, for example, Secretary of Health and Human Services Otis Bowen wrote to six Republican senators to assure that no federal funds were being spent for research on RU-486 as an abortifacient. Instead, he said, NIH scientists were studying the drug in "projects related to breast cancer, lymphoma, glaucoma, Cushing's syndrome, basic reproductive biology and its potential use as a contraceptive." He added that scientists elsewhere were exploring its possible use in AIDS research.

A few months later, in a letter seeking support for a bill prohibiting the use of federal funds in research on RU-486, Congressman Robert Dornan of California labeled it, "the death pill." He distorted our early clinical results, and concluded, "The taking of a pre-born life will be as easy and as trivial as taking aspirin."

With its proven record elsewhere, the fate of RU-486 in America rests on the political will of its supporters. The problem posed is not whether RU-486 is a safe medical alternative for women seeking to exercise their legal right to abortion, but whether activists can keep them from exercising that right.

The answer should be simple. No one should be permitted to intrude on a woman's decision to terminate a pregnancy. That right of privacy has been upheld by the U.S. Supreme Court. In a system defined by the U.S. Constitution, such moral judgments can only be forced upon others by elected legislators. If a medical procedure is legal, and people want to use it, objectors can only object.

As undistorted facts reached more people, new forces gathered to bolster RU-486's original champions. The bullying tactics of anti-abortionists began to disgust many Americans, whatever their stand on the issue.

At the end of 1990, RU-486 was on the cover of *New Republic*. There was a full-sized portrait, a little white pill in the center of the cover under the headline "Miracle Drug." Underneath, a bold caption read: "When RU-486, the French abortion pill, was just a safe way to end pregnancy, anti-abortion activists had little trouble keeping it out of the country. Now doctors say the drug also promises to be a breakthrough treatment for brain tumors, breast cancer, Cushing's syndrome and even infertility—and the pro-life movement has a problem."

Along with political will in America, RU-486 will need a push from its manufacturer. In 1991, moves began in that direction. Edouard Sakiz met with George Zeidenstein, president of the Population Council, to breathe new life into the 1982 agreement, which allows the council to organize abortion trials in the United States, and, after FDA approval, permits public non-profit organizations to distribute it.

If large-scale trials are undertaken as expected, there are a range of options. Even if Roussel-Uclaf itself chooses not to market its product in the United States, family planning groups and potential investors are anxious to play some role. RU-486 will make its American entrance: science, good sense, and freedom will triumph.

RU-486's place in America must be seen not only in a broad social setting but also its historical context. The regulations are hardly new. No laws restricted abortion in 1800, and many women suffered. In the early days, the problem was not morality but the limits of medical science. By 1900, after a century of tumultuous debate, it was outlawed practically everywhere. And women continued to suffer.

In a book entitled *Abortion in America*, James Mohr, professor of history at the University of Maryland, traces how the question evolved during the crucial nineteenth century.

Until the 1800s, only British common law applied to abortion in America. A fetus was protected after "quickening," when the woman could feel its first movements late in the fourth month or early in the fifth. After that, abortion was considered a crime, but not a serious one. The issue was the mother's welfare, not the destruction of a human being.

No reliable pregnancy tests existed; quickening was the only clear clue. A doctor, or the woman herself, could take measures to remove an unnatural "blockage" of menstruation. The same means as for performing an abortion were used. The moral issue of whether a fetus was alive had gone unresolved for five thousand years, Mohr observed, and no one belabored the question.

In 1803, the British Parliament made abortion before quickening a criminal offense. No American state took similar action. In a tolerant climate, some American doctors applied their growing knowledge to performing abortions, but this was not common. Instead, home medical manuals suggested ways to provoke miscarriage, including bloodletting and strong punches to the belly. Indian herbal healers were in vogue, with such remedies as myrrh, aloe, and snakeroot.

Abortion was sought mostly by single women, often from respectable families, who wanted to keep their pregnancy secret. It was not seen as a means of family planning. The practice, Mohr wrote, "was neither morally nor legally wrong in the eyes of the vast majority of Americans, provided it was accomplished before quickening."

A Connecticut law in 1821 barred anyone from giving poisons to a pregnant woman after quickening. It said nothing about mechanical or surgical means, nor about noxious substances before quickening. Only the practitioner, not the patient, was punished. In 1830, the statute was broadened to cover abortion by any means. But in deliberate separation from English law, abortion before quickening remained legal.

The fight in the United States was over regulating medicine; abortion was a side issue. During Colonial times, doctors with formal degrees had social standing but were not particularly skillful. When a new democracy broke down old barriers, others sought to take their place. By the early 1800s, anyone could claim the title of doctor. Practiced free-lancers, quacks, and folk healers all competed with "regular" doctors who had studied in medical schools. This not only eroded the physicians' standing but also cut into their earnings.

The "regulars" tended to shun abortion. Their creed was the Hippocratic Oath and, unlike Plato and Socrates, Hippocrates opposed abortion. Many regulars were distressed by the damage of incompetent abortions. Others saw themselves losing patients to "irregulars," who were prepared to offer a service demanded widely among women.

Doctors trained in science generally rejected quickening as a meaningless point of reference. They saw fetal development as a continuous process. If abortion was wrong after quickening, they argued, then it could also be wrong before.

During the early 1800s, physicians began to form medical associations to further their science—and to defend their interests. Their strongest arm was the law, and they lobbied intensely in state legislatures.

"The first wave of abortion legislation in American history emerged from the struggles of . . . legislators and physicians to control medical practice rather than from public pressure to deal with abortion per se," Mohr notes. None of the laws passed between 1821 and 1841 punished the woman. "All of this reflected the continued perception of abortion in the United States as a fundamentally marginal practice usually resorted to by women who deserved pity and protection rather than criminal liability."

In the 1840s, abortion moved into the public view. White Protestant women of respectable families seized on it as a way to limit childbearing. The number of abortions soared and, suddenly, they were big business. "Madame Restell," an English immigrant, opened shop in New York and soon had branches in Boston and Philadelphia. Her salesmen hawked abortifacient pills on the road. Periodic arrests and convictions on minor counts only bolstered her fame and fueled her publicity over thirty-five years.

Madame Restell made the headlines. By 1871, she had reportedly spent $60,000 expanding not only her own share but also the whole market. "CAUTION—No 'Female Monthly Pills' are genuine except those sold at Madame Restell's principal office," warned one advertisement. It referred to the wave of "counterfeits and imitations" advertised widely in newspapers eager for the ad revenue. In one week in 1845, the *Boston Daily*

Times carried five ads, including those for Madame Drunette's French Lunar Pills and Dr. Peter's French Renovating Pills, "sure to produce a miscarriage."

All of this provoked sharp reaction among regular doctors. E. P. Le Prohon, a Frenchman who settled in New England, wrote that the ads corrupted children, who understood them as well as parents did. The increase in abortions could be traced to "the dissemination of immoral and criminal advertisements in daily journals," he said. But outrage was limited.

In 1860, quickening remained the determining point of pregnancy. Thirteen of the thirty-three American states still had no abortion laws.

An organization set up in 1847 eventually made the difference: the American Medical Association. Horatio Storer, a young gynecologist from Boston, rallied physicians to his cause. After the AMA's 1859 meeting in Louisville, Kentucky, the fast-growing association led the fight to outlaw abortion in the United States. Storer fought for federal laws. Some colleagues also wanted to condemn abortifacient suppliers and advertisers, but he decided not to test the AMA's strength against drug manufacturers.

The AMA was hardly unanimous. A large minority argued that women should not be put at risk to save unborn fetuses. But Storer's arguments carried. Doctors felt that abortions, as practiced then, were too great a medical risk. And they also were eager to turn the law on the interlopers—"irregulars" they regarded as incompetent—in a profession they sought to police.

This campaign by medical specialists undermined the traditional tolerance for abortion in America. An issue that had been dismissed as unimportant, and in dubious taste, was now openly debated. Fledgling feminist organizations weighed in, surprisingly mostly against abortion. They saw it as manipulation by males to dominate female sexuality. Instead of forcing abortion on women, they argued, men should practice abstinence.

Religious leaders gave only tepid support to the AMA. The Protestant clergy were uncomfortable discussing sexuality. Many church leaders agreed with their congregations that no moral issue arose: a fetus was not alive before quickening. Since most women seeking abortions were Protestant, ministers chose not to interfere.

Bishop Fitzpatrick of Boston hailed the AMA campaign, but it was ten years before Roman Catholic leaders spoke out again. A council of bishops in Baltimore condemned all abortions, including therapeutic abortion advocated by the AMA.

Mohr concluded: "Although American churchmen certainly did not oppose the anti-abortion crusade, neither did they become conspicuously involved in it, especially compared to their involvement in various other nineteenth-century movements for the alteration of social policy, such as temperance."

By 1900, abortion was illegal across the United States. Madame Restell, finally arrested on felony charges in 1878, had committed suicide before trial. Married Protestant women had begun to reject the practice. Abortion returned to back alleys, largely a final resort for poor, desperate women until, in 1973, the Supreme Court ruled in favor of an anonymous Texas woman whom legal documents named Jane Roe.

In *Roe v. Wade*, the court defined the limits of state regulation of abortion. Roughly speaking, in the first trimester, the decision to have an abortion lies with the woman and her doctor. In the second trimester, states may regulate the abortion procedure in ways reasonably related to the mother's health. In the third trimester, states may prohibit abortion except where necessary to the health of the mother.

If it legalized abortion in the United States, the *Roe* decision also galvanized a right-to-life movement which up until then had lacked a rallying point. Patient, persistent campaigning put sympathetic people in state legislatures and on the bench. The law was clear, but public attitudes were mixed. In 1966, as unbelievable as it may be, contraception still was illegal in Massachusetts even among married couples.

The election of President Reagan in 1980 fired new enthusiasm into the anti-abortion campaign. Reagan left no doubt about his stand. In one address, his voice catching with emotion, he pronounced that a human life began at conception. He declared January 17, 1988, as National Sanctity of Human Life Day, dedicated to protecting the unborn.

Reagan's proclamation noted the "tragic and unspeakable" loss of "22 million infants" since *Roe v. Wade*, which was the total of legal abortions. He evoked the "pressure and anguish of countless women and girls who are driven to abortion." However, he ignored what would have happened, in terms of lost lives and women's anguish, had abortion not been legal.

At Reagan's request, Surgeon General Everett Koop made a detailed study on abortion in America. Though against abortion, Koop was bound by principle to take a professional view. In January 1989, he reported that he had found no medical or psychological reason to condemn the practice.

The administration resisted *Roe v. Wade* whenever possible, sometimes with tragic results. The Centers for Disease Control in Atlanta prepared guidelines for counseling women exposed to AIDS on how to avoid transmitting the virus to children. Although over one in ten babies born to AIDS-infected women die before they are five, the CDC neglected to mention abortion as an option. Sick children suffer delirium, pain, convulsions, and paralysis.

The Reagan administration not only froze federal funds for any research or family planning centers smacking of abortion but also cut off aid to international agencies or foreign national programs with the slightest connection to abortion. This crippled desperately needed family planning in the Third World.

Today, a glance at television or newspapers is enough to suggest the virulence of the debate. Hundreds of thousands of people throng downtown Washington for or against abortion. In small Midwestern towns, police need billy clubs to separate zealots on either side. Self-appointed vigilantes prevent women from keeping appointments at abortion clinics. At one Ohio clinic, a defender of choice plowed into protesters with his pickup truck.

As a result, political campaigns can be swayed by the abortion issue. When the Idaho legislature passed a repressive law, people around the country swore off Idaho potatoes. The governor vetoed the law, to thunderous reaction from both sides. At each opening on the Supreme Court, the burning question is how a candidate sees *Roe v. Wade*. Pressure groups in opposing camps leap upon any public sampling which seems to support its particular position. In 1990, a Louis Harris poll reported that 73 percent of American adults believe a woman should choose for herself. This only spurred on the anti-abortionists.

As might be expected, in the United States news of RU-486 arrived like a splash of gasoline on a blazing fire. At Roussel-Uclaf, a basement storeroom is lined with cardboard file boxes marked *pour* and *contre*. My own files bulge with the same sort of letters. There are pleas and diatribes, petitions and threats. A few propose me for prizes; another starts out, "Piece of manure!" One tells me, "I want you to know that my family (consisting of two daughters, five nieces, husbands, fathers and grandparents) all applaud your research."

It is tempting to total up those for and against, but the numbers would be skewed. I noticed one letter that began, "Dear Mr. Uclaf." It urged that the company stop "testing, marketing and distributing" the product "anywhere in the world." Then I found dozens of others, all variations peppered with the exact same expressions. Similar series showed up, both for and against. Some were identical computer-generated letters with different signatures.

Here was the phenomenon of American lobbying at work. How many times have I seen it? "Dear Member, Enclosed is a letter to be sent . . . We suggest that you vary the wording so it does not appear . . ." What results is not a sampling of public opinion but rather a measure of one or another side's ability to marshal its forces.

A careful reading of the letters reveals that what disturbs people about RU-486 is primarily abortion itself. Many are from the heart, inspired by nothing but the writers' reaction to something that is important to them. A man in small-town Texas, "being a former embryo/fetus myself," asked that the pill be scrapped. A woman in Castorland, New York, wrote, "This product will not help our world but destroy it."

Most detractors were badly misinformed about the pill, but

their vehemence rattled some European executives used to
milder discourse. One couple wrote, "What a horrible world we
live in if people can just abort the lives of unborn babies by
popping a pill in their mouths. What an *evil evil* company you
must be to produce and distribute such a murderous weapon."
A lot of letters have a feel that is ugly beyond the content.
One, scrawled in blue ballpoint on lined yellow paper, pronounced in underlined words: "We will not allow its marketing
here in the United States. End production of RU-486 now." The
last word was underlined three times, in hard, jabbing strokes.
    There was some toughness on the other side, too. The
president of a state chapter of NOW wrote: "Please bring RU-
486 to the U.S. Don't fear a boycott from the anti-abortionists.
You should fear a boycott from us if you don't help keep abortion
safe, legal, affordable and accessible in the U.S."
    Some were angry, such as one that lamented that "Cather-
ine the Great of Russia, Cleopatra VII of Egypt, and Eleanor of
Aquitaine" were not around to replace men as leaders of the
world. Addressed to Edouard Sakiz, it ended: "Take heed, cowardly little man, the great women will return." Another wrote:
"RU-486 is the 'moral property of ALL women,' not just those
who are fortunate enough to be able to fly to France. My body is
not the property of the Roman Catholic Church or President
Bush. Abortion has been around since ancient times, and it is
very unethical of Roussel-Uclaf to hoard the technology of this
revolutionary pill. . . . I am sure if RU-486 proves effective in
treating prostate cancer a lot of men will change their minds."
    Some were from highly placed people. Jo Ann Zimmerman,
a former obstetrical nurse, wrote on her letterhead as lieutenant
governor of Iowa: "I do not want to return to the kind of health
care available to women before . . . *Roe v. Wade*. . . . Women
have continued to gain in controlling our own reproductive destiny. RU-486 is a positive move for women to continue controlling their choice of when to carry a pregnancy." The president of
the American Pediatric Society praised the pill, emphasizing the
group's belief that every child has the right to be wanted.
    I was moved most by simple, handwritten pleas which

showed me that women in America had understood what was being offered to them. "I am writing to implore your influence in promoting the sale of the drug RU-486 in the United States," began one to Sakiz from a woman in New Jersey. "If there are medical advances that can benefit women, it is not fair to deny them to us. The people who believe abortion is murder do not speak for me and should not be able to prevent me from having one. . . . Again, I implore you to help provide RU-486 to American women."

Letters to Roussel-Uclaf eventually end up with Ariel Mouttet, who oversees the product's passage abroad. Normally, she replies with a brief form letter, and the correspondence ends. One morning in July 1990 she walked into company headquarters to find the spacious lobby filled with cardboard crates stenciled with her name. A ten-person American delegation had flown to Paris to urge importation of the pill. They brought 125,000 signatures on petitions, one thousand pounds of documents.

The group included Carl Djerassi, whose work enabled Pincus to proceed toward the oral contraceptive, Myron Allukian, Jr., president of the American Public Health Association, and Eleanor Smeal, president of the Feminist Majority Foundation and former NOW president. They spent the morning with Sakiz. He was already persuaded, he told them. Their target was in Frankfurt. The committee loaded their half-ton of names into a Roussel truck and moved on to Hoechst. There they did not change anyone's mind.

Roussel-Uclaf products are normally marketed in the United States by Hoechst-Roussel Pharmaceuticals Inc., 20 percent of which is owned by the French partner. The remainder is controlled by Hoechst Celanese Corporation, the German partner's main American subsidiary. Hoechst Celanese's $6 billion annual sales—for everything from tires to textiles—account for nearly a quarter of Hoechst A.G.'s worldwide earnings. The German-American firm does not like RU-486 at all.

Each company has its own corporate policy. HRPI does not sell fertility control products, but Roussel has its own American subsidiary which could handle a company product like RU-486. Other corporate structures could be devised with outside interests. In any situation, Hoechst has the determining vote.

Fear of a boycott is only part of the picture. The huge German company is sensitive to consumer pressure, but it could wait out any resistance that the anti-abortionists might organize. In his book *Abortion: The Clash of Absolutes*, Harvard law professor Lawrence Tribe recalls a similar threat to makers of oral contraceptives. Searle pioneered the market by ignoring the threatened boycott. Parke-Davis Group, which backed out, lost heavily. More recently, Upjohn Company dropped prostaglandin research. The company reported that a threatened boycott had no measurable effect. It acted because of a problem that profoundly worries Hoechst: liability.

In the ruthlessly litigious climate of the United States, the pharmaceutical industry is very sensitive, especially in the field of reproductive medicine.

In the early 1970s, a popular intrauterine device called the Dalkon Shield rivaled the pill. Soon, complaints of infections rolled in. Its manufacturer, A. H. Robins Company, hid the facts. After 320,000 claims were filed, the court stepped in. Before Robins sank into bankruptcy, the company was ordered to put aside $2.475 billion for settlements.

The punitive judgments were understandable. The Dalkon Shield caused serious, sometimes fatal infections because it was badly designed. Like the tragic case of thalidomide, liability was clear-cut. Even before the Dalkon Shield scandal, however, there was the experience of Depo-Provera, an efficient and safe injectable contraceptive developed by Upjohn.

In 1974, the FDA had decided to approve Depo-Provera as a contraceptive. The drug was also being used to treat certain cases of breast cancer. A campaign by feminists who cited disagreeable side effects prompted the FDA to demur. After spending an estimated $100 million on the project, Upjohn backed away. Today, Depo-Provera is distributed widely elsewhere in the world but not in the United States.

In the field of reproduction, spontaneous anomalies can

throw unfounded suspicion on medicine. Even when a company is blameless, lawsuits drain resources and reputation. Liability insurance is difficult to get. Drug makers, who have seen the effect of an aroused American public, prefer a simple response: "We don't operate in that field."

Not one large American pharmaceutical company has expressed interest in taking up Roussel-Uclaf's patent. Except for the Ortho Pharmaceutical Corporation, a division of Johnson & Johnson, they have all but abandoned research in birth control over the past twenty years. Since 1980, eight major companies dropped out of the contraceptive field.

A two-year study by the National Research Council and the Institute of Medicine blamed not only product liability laws but also restrictive regulations and a lack of public research funds. Three specialists reporting their findings in *The New England Journal of Medicine* in 1990, wrote: "The nation offers far more support for research to alleviate specific illnesses than to prevent the burdens and trauma of unwanted pregnancy and its medical, psychological and social consequences." And they concluded: "Unless immediate steps are taken to change public policy, the choice of contraceptives in the United States in the next century will not differ appreciably from what it is today."

One of the authors was Luigi Mastroianni, professor of obstetrics and gynecology at the University of Pennsylvania. At a news conference on the report, he stressed the aspect of liability which blocks medical advances ready to be marketed. He said:

"While we in the United States make do with the same range of options available thirty years ago, in some European countries people can choose among contraceptive implants, injectable contraceptives, and a variety of pills, IUDs and sterilization techniques not available here."

Also in 1990, Djerassi wrote in *Science* magazine, "The United States is the only country other than Iran in which the birth-control clock has been set backward during the past decade." In a twist of irony, the chemist who helped pioneer the pill suggested in the article that people again think about using the good old fallible rhythm method.

In this atmosphere, reluctance in the Hoechst group is easy to understand. There are also commercial reasons. HRPI has no experience in marketing drugs for reproductive control. It would need a new network for sales, distribution, and control. Licensing RU-486 would require at least $70 million for clinical testing and meeting other FDA requirements. Large provisions would have to be set aside to weather consumer protests.

For Hoechst directors, other fears have little to do with profits. They understand the weapons of a "down and dirty fight." Activists have called on Nazi ghosts before, however much Germany has since been transformed. Here was the same problem again. With such a risk and no glory, what is the motivation? There is social responsibility, but who is to define that?

RU-486's constituency in America has grown steadily as more people insist on simple reason. People need it and want it. There is no legal or medical obstacle. Across a broad social spectrum, a clear majority supports a woman's right to abortion. Those people who oppose abortion can shun RU-486. But they should not be allowed to keep it from others.

Once scientists develop the other potentials of RU-486, the drug can be put to use against maladies unrelated to fertility control. It may well save the lives of some of those people who now insist that it is a death pill.

In the face of an American groundswell, Hoechst and Roussel-Uclaf may soon find a way to act. They own the patent. If they don't use it, they can share it or cede it. On the French side, there are strong, justifiable feelings of pride. Their product has proved itself. Why shouldn't its flag fly in the United States?

Among the medical and scientific communities, attitudes toward RU-486 are increasingly positive. Some specialists express frustration, even hostility, at not being able to get enough RU-486 for work they want to do.

By the time RU-486 became available in France, American scientists knew it well. When a drug is not licensed for commercial use, the FDA allows scientific imports under an IND, an investigational new drug permit. The Population Council obtained an IND and arranged for clinical trials, importing RU-486 under the agreement it had signed with Roussel-Uclaf. At the University of Southern California Women's Hospital in Los Angeles, doctors performed abortions and reported up to 90 percent success by using RU-486 alone, without prostaglandin.

Other scientific groups imported the drug, either through the Population Council or with INDs they had obtained on their own. Roussel-Uclaf made RU-486 available to researchers in a number of fields, but controversy began to interfere.

In 1987, after three years, the Population Council stopped its support for the USC trials. *Mother Jones* magazine reported later that the council was pressured by powerful people, including Senator Jesse Helms of North Carolina. The article pointed out how vulnerable scientists can be to political influences. "There are other ways a researcher can be pressured besides just having money cut off for a particular project," Wayne Bardin, the council's director of medical research, was quoted as saying. "You can have money blocked for some other research you want to do." If not for pressure, he said, "RU-486 would really be a number one priority."

Daniel Mishell, chairman of obstetrics and gynecology at USC, remained enthusiastic and continued with the work. But in February 1990 the program abruptly stopped. The supply of RU-486 ran out after four hundred doses. David Grimes, Mishell's associate, blamed Roussel-Uclaf for not providing more.

Under the circumstances, everyone's maneuvering room was limited. Roussel-Uclaf, which had to answer to Hoechst, insisted that INDs for abortion trials be channeled only through the Population Council, according to the 1982 agreement. Bardin said that he could not raise funds to support RU-486 research because Roussel's plans were so unclear. "Until Roussel makes a decision, there is nothing to say," he observed in early 1991.

A group of doctors at the University of California in San Francisco, led by Bernard Gore, sought to organize new trials with RU-486. They applied to the Population Council and Roussel-Uclaf for the drug. Neither produced any.

Although Roussel had given large amounts of the drug to researchers working in fields outside of fertility control, there were inevitable conflicts. A number of scientists and specialists wanted to experiment with RU-486 on various medical grounds. The company did not want to overextend its exposure.

During 1990, the issue erupted in Washington. Though banned from abortion research, NIH scientists made headway in other areas. Suddenly some supplies of RU-486 were stopped. Scientists elsewhere complained that research was at risk. Congressman Ron Wyden, a Democrat from Oregon, called a hearing of the House Subcommittee on Regulation, Business Opportunities, and Energy.

Newspapers, especially *The Washington Post*, reported at length on the sometimes stormy proceedings over the French pill.

Wyden accused the FDA of bending to Bush administration prejudice, causing "needless suffering" to Americans. The ban, he said, was "arbitrary, political, and unscientific."

FDA counsel Sandra Barnes countered that the FDA "has no choice but to enforce a statute—which Congress has not seen fit to change." In fact, added Ronald Chesemore, associate commissioner for regulatory affairs, agency officials "place no restrictions on research." I agree: it was all a mistake.

Along with INDs, the FDA may grant permission for individuals to import small amounts of an unlicensed drug for personal use. Because of the controversy—some charged because of official pressure—the FDA canceled personal importation of RU-486. Chesemore said that researchers were inadvertently misled when the FDA issued an "import alert" to prohibit personal use.

At times, the hearing became a public trial of RU-486. "I am a practicing Catholic who is unalterably opposed to abortion," said Helen Byrne, a breast cancer victim and vice president of the Cancer Patients Action Alliance (CANACT). "But the issue here is not abortion. The issue is life or death of women with breast cancer."

The problem, Wyden said, was that the FDA's personal import ban created a climate of regulatory "resistance" when it should be "an active advocate" for medical research. As a result, he said, Roussel-Uclaf has made it difficult or impossible for U.S. researchers to be reliably supplied with RU-486.

An American Medical Association statement said the FDA had acted responsibly. Other witnesses said the agency was caught in the middle; the fault was with the company, which did not seek to license its drug or encourage researchers to use it.

Wyden demanded to know what the FDA would do "to turn this situation around." Why couldn't it get Health and Human Services chief Louis W. Sullivan to call Roussel-Uclaf? Chesemore, barely masking his exasperation, replied: "It is not in the authority of the FDA to make corporate decisions."

In fact, the FDA did what it should have done. Personal importation had never been envisioned; RU-486 use should be supervised by a doctor following the appropriate protocol. The FDA can issue INDs only with the approval of the manufacturer. The Population Council had rights to import RU-486. Otherwise, it was up to Roussel. The company had a right to decide whose research was likely to produce results.

The primary problem was Hoechst's opposition. That was beyond the reach of American authorities.

Meanwhile, in publications and at meetings, doctors demanded with growing vehemence that RU-486 be made available. They argued that a nonscientific fringe should not be allowed to suppress it.

In August 1990, the *Journal of the American Medical Association* carried a commentary by William Regelson, Roger Loria, and Mohammed Kalimi which concluded: "If Hoechst-Roussel cannot resist threats of boycott, then the rights to study or commercially develop mifepristone should be assigned to focused groups not subject to economic pressure. The value of mifepristone must be decided by physicians in the clinical arena. It is time to join the public debate on the ethics of denying drugs to the living because of political activism regarding the unborn."

Regelson, an oncologist at the Medical College of Virginia, observed elsewhere, "If RU-486 did not have abortion associated with it, it would be considered a major breakthrough drug."

The *JAMA* article reviewed RU-486's potential to medicine, and it concluded: "Unfortunately, the political and economic consequences of the threatened anti-abortion boycott . . . have largely frozen clinical trials. . . . If abortion remains a legal option, the availability of mifepristone must be decided by clinical data and not on the basis of economic threats by those who are opposed on ethical or religious grounds. The emotionalism of this issue threatens all future clinical research with antiprogestins or glucocorticoid receptor blockers. . . . It is tragic that in this country 43,000 victims die of breast cancer each year, while abject surrender to abortion politics delays clinical studies that might help them."

RU-486 is not the miracle drug for cancer; its effectiveness has been proven in a number of cases not significant enough to draw conclusions, and is still being explored. But the article reflected a deepening concern among American scientists.

Professional associations took clear positions in favor of RU-486. The American Association for the Advancement of Science, which groups specialists of all disciplines, added its support.

In June 1990, the American Medical Association, in a resounding vote, supported the "legal availability of RU-486 for appropriate research and, if indicated, clinical practice." The AMA, which had come into existence in the nineteenth century opposing abortion because of its dangers, was now championing a method to make it safer and showing that its interest was medical, not ideological.

RU-486 has built a particularly strong following among the women who would use it. Early in 1989, when 300,000 to 500,000 people gathered in Washington for a "march for women's lives," the largest political demonstration in American history, the crowd roared approval when speakers mentioned the molecule.

The Planned Parenthood Federation of America rallied around RU-486 from the start. PPFA has grown into the forward-thinking, sensitive organization envisioned by Margaret Sanger, and its medical personnel have expertly countered the arguments of misinformed anti-abortionists. Its dynamic president, Faye

Wattleton, has made three trips to Paris to plead with Roussel-Uclaf.

The National Organization for Women, the National Abortion Rights Action League, the Fund for the Feminist Majority, and other groups lent their support. A number of specialized groups also took up the banner: Henry David's Transnational Family Research Institute, Malcolm Potts's Family Health International, the Population Crisis Committee, the Alan Guttmacher Institute, and the American Health Foundation, among others. We were helped by exceptional women who worked on their own for the pill, such as Deeda Blair, Robin Chandler Duke, and Joanne Woodward. Rebecca Cook, a law professor at the University of Toronto, taught us the legal questions operating in different countries.

I was especially encouraged by support from women's organizations. While anti-abortionists took it upon themselves to speak for God and unborn infants, women were speaking about their own lives.

Press comment in the United States reflects a strong public feeling that Americans want Roussel-Uclaf to take a stand. Editorials were heavily in favor of RU-486 from the beginning.

In March 1988, *The New York Times* noted, "Clearly, then, there is an American market for RU-486. Now, where's the marketeer?" That spring, others echoed that thought. The *Philadelphia Inquirer* called for more courage from the U.S. government and the French manufacturer. *The Washington Post* urged that RU-486 be brought to America.

When the storm first broke, the *Boston Globe* wrote, "An all-out effort is needed to win release of the abortion pill RU-486 into the international medical community." In 1990, in an editorial entitled "A Pill Whose Time Has Come," the *Globe* added, "The advantages of RU-486 are so clear-cut that it cannot long be denied to American women . . . the ultimate reason is, as the French health minister says, that this drug is 'the moral property' of all women."

And *The New York Times* came back with a broader message: "Getting RU-486 more widely distributed will take a humane, worldwide effort that would benefit from leadership by, and in, the United States."

Vanity Fair magazine highlighted the pill in an article, in 1989, which made an important point: "Already, the anti-abortionists have acknowledged that the new drug could complicate their task. 'We're really very simplistic, visually oriented people,' Dr. John Willke of the National Right to Life Committee told one reporter. 'And if what [abortions] destroy in there doesn't look human, then it will make our job much more difficult.' "

Willke and the others, of course, were not daunted. Anti-abortion zealots campaigned with loaded words. RU-486 was the chemical coat hanger. It was the Dalkon Shield of the '90s. I was a mass murderer. Periodically, researchers connected with the drug received anonymous death threats. More than anything else, I found this paradoxical.

But the right-to-life position was hardly funny, in light of reality. Deaths dropped sharply when abortion came out of hiding. Women still die each year, and many more suffer permanent damage.

In the name of morality, anti-abortionists block aid to poor mothers who desperately need access to safe abortion. They oppose RU-486, which can broaden the options and lower costs.

Medicine needs all the tools that science can offer. Yet right-to-life crusaders distort facts that contest their point of view. In ignorance or in malice, they deny evidence of RU-486's potential in treating disease.

Much of the serious opposition to RU-486 in America bases itself on religion. It is hardly clear-cut, however. As time has gone on, support has begun to crystallize among some church leaders who had reserved judgment during the early controversy.

Too often, in the United States and elsewhere, the abortion issue is seen as between "the church" on the one side and undefined liberals on the other. The Roman Catholic Church declares that abortion is murder, based on the tenet that a person begins at fertilization. In fact, that position dates only from 1869.

Fundamentalist sects that take a similar position have no text to cite.

Neither Protestants, nor Jews, nor Moslems, nor the principal Asian religions—not even Orthodox Catholics—insist that an embryo of a few days is sacred. Some faiths fix a time later in the continuum when a soul enters the fetus to form a new human being. Others leave it up to an individual's conscience. Although most religions generally oppose abortion, several allow such contragestive methods as menstrual regulation.

As right-to-life activists raised their tone against RU-486, several churches began to speak out. Late in 1990, Sakiz received a letter from Charles Shelby Rooks, executive vice president of the United Church Board for Homeland Ministries. The board oversees domestic missions of the United Church of Christ, a bedrock Protestant denomination which counts 1.5 million members and traces its roots to the Pilgrims and early German reformers.

The board voted to support further tests of RU-486, after which they would back its distribution, Rooks reported. "The directors saw their vote for further testing as a logical step in their affirmation of women as moral agents," he wrote. "The directors find it deeply distressful that a group of our citizens would deny a woman a less invasive method of terminating a pregnancy and deny humankind the benefit of further research that could lead to more effective treatment of cancer, glaucoma and endometriosis. The directors also find it deeply distressing that when five hundred women a day are dying of botched surgical abortions, this potentially life-saving alternative is being blocked by a few people."

Among Catholics, who make up 26 percent of the U.S. population, the issue is complex. The Vatican's position against abortion is unequivocal. Yet 32 percent of abortions in America are performed on Catholic women.

Archbishop Rembert Weakland of Milwaukee conducted "listening sessions" on abortion, earning him reproof from Rome but praise from many Catholics. "Archbishop Weakland, who clearly supports the church's teachings on abortion, has worked to create rational discourse with those who disagree," wrote *Conscience*, the journal of Catholics for a Free Choice.

Turmoil around Governor Mario Cuomo of New York brought the Catholic dilemma into sharp focus in 1990. After Cuomo refused to seek a ban on abortion, Bishop Austin Vaughan of Albany suggested in public that he was headed to hell. A New York City bishop refused to allow him to speak in diocesan institutions. In the *New York Review of Books*, late in 1990, Garry Wills recalled how Cuomo had defined his ground in a 1984 speech at Notre Dame University after John Cardinal O'Connor refused to condemn those who demanded his excommunication.

The Catholic Church influences American politics along two tracks, Wills noted. Its own members are expected to follow its doctrine. On the second track, "It addresses outsiders, 'men [*sic*] of good will,' with well-formulated arguments from a long natural-law tradition." Such measures as voluntary codes in films, for example, are not presented as religious matters but rather as a defense of civil decency.

Cuomo told the gathering at Notre Dame that while he personally banned abortion as it applied to his own family, he was bound to uphold the laws he was elected to administer. But more, he described the ambivalence many Catholics felt toward the Church's position. In a carefully worded passage, Cuomo asked:

"Despite the teaching in our homes and schools and pulpits, despite the sermons and pleadings of parents and priests and prelates, despite all the effort at defining our opposition to the sin of abortion, collectively we Catholics apparently believe—and perhaps act—little differently from those who don't share our commitment. Are we asking government to make criminal what we believe to be sinful because we ourselves can't stop committing the sin?"

In his own analysis, Wills noted the deep divisions among Catholics. Neither contraception nor the origin of the soul is mentioned in the scriptures; they have been discussed in various ways in successive papal decrees over the centuries. The Church's second track of influence—moral persuasion based on the natural-law tradition—is all the weaker for lack of clear definition of "natural law."

On the issue of abortion and birth control, even many devout believers questioned the Church's authority. "Most Catholics," Wills observed, "have concluded that their clerical leaders are unhinged on the subject of sex."

In 1989, the Supreme Court's *Webster v. Reproductive Health Services* decision provided new openings for the right-to-life movement. The *Webster* decision allowed states to block public funds for abortion. It upheld a Missouri statute that declares that "the life of each human being begins at conception." It suggested that the Court might be edging toward a reversal of *Roe v. Wade.* The decision, in effect, invited state legislatures to enact more restrictive abortion laws.

Under the Missouri law, doctors could be obliged to do fetus viability tests before an abortion after the twenty-second week. The murkily worded text made no medical sense; twenty-two weeks is clearly too early for any fetus to survive outside the womb. Such tests might endanger the mother or the fetus. The law amounted to a means of discouraging abortions for women needing public assistance, mostly poor and often young and black. Mid-1991, anti-abortionists launched a campaign of violence and made Wichita, Kansas, a first target. The Louisiana state legislature passed an abortion law so restrictive that its purpose was clearly to challenge *Roe v. Wade* before a new Supreme Court. In June, a new judge, David Souter, cast the swing vote in upholding a ban on abortion counseling in federally funded clinics. Then Justice Thurgood Marshall retired, leaving his seat to a conservative. Abortion seemed headed for a serious test in court.

Webster, however, had the unintended effect of demonstrating the anti-abortionists' weakness in state legislatures. Of more than 350 bills to restrict abortion put forward by the end of 1990, only Pennsylvania, South Carolina, West Virginia, Utah, and Guam passed laws. A few states followed in 1991, but others went in the opposite direction. Remarkably, New Hampshire

offered itself for large-scale abortion trials of RU-486. At the
same time many legislators rallied behind free choice, which
many saw as a popular cause. Both the House and Senate approved bills that would permit doctors to advise women on abortion in all family planning centers. The President would have to
use his veto to stop Congress from reversing the Supreme Court.

Public figures found their statements scrutinized by both
sides. When someone asked Marilyn Quayle, wife of the Vice
President, what should be done for women made pregnant by
rape, she replied: "Something like the French morning-after pill
would be very appropriate." Damage-control statements quickly
followed, explaining that was not what she meant.

In the new climate, some cracks opened in the solid front
left over from the Reagan days. Three women made waves by
resigning from the New York State Republican Finance Committee when they could not convince party leaders to soften their
stand on abortion. Barbara Gimbel, Barbara Mossbacher, and
Pauline Harrison took up the pro-choice banner after the *Webster*
decision. They led what one magazine called the "White-Glove
Brigade."

They scored major points. Republican party national chairman Lee Atwater announced that the GOP had room for more
than one position on abortion. The women argued that a policy
shift was essential for the party's survival. Mrs. Harrison cited a
poll that indicated 92 percent of New York State voters favored
free choice. "You can't ignore those political facts anymore," she
told a reporter. "These people who don't support us are a minority of radicals, I would say. The mind-set of any radical is a
strange one."

Mrs. Mossbacher invited me to New York to speak on RU-
486 at a Republican party fund raiser. After all that Reagan's
government had done to stop abortion at home and around the
world, the party would be raising money on my name. The
electoral platform of the New York Republican party has since
become pro-choice. The idea of mixing politics with family planning displeases me, but I was delighted to see this softening
stand.

Attitudes were also shifting among leaders in the black community. Years ago, many American blacks believed that birth control and abortion were cunning means to keep them in their demographic minority. Since Martin Luther King, that position has changed. King, honored in 1966 by Planned Parenthood, commented that Margaret Sanger "launched a movement that is obeying a higher law to preserve human life under human conditions." It is poor single mothers of any race who are most in need of protection from unwanted childbearing.

And as RU-486 gained fame, Mayor David Dinkins of New York joined other black leaders to speak out for it. Early in 1991, he told a Planned Parenthood conference: "Today I declare to you my intention to spearhead a group of mayors in the effort to make RU-486 available in the United States by creating a 'safe climate' for the import, testing, and eventual distribution of better and safer means of reproductive control."

Dinkins took up the banner, not as a black leader, but as mayor of the nation's largest city. He kept his promise to rally other mayors around the country. And he wrote to Sakiz with a lesson in American politics that helped to convince Roussel officials that the mood was changing: "Why allow a small minority to frustrate the large majority by the use of, as lawyers call it, a 'heckler's veto'—i.e., when one heckler ruins a speech for all? Lonely hecklers should be ignored."

Dinkins proposed a possible "risk pool" at a federal level to encourage drug companies to brave product-liability suits. He also volunteered New York as a base for action on behalf of RU-486. American law guaranteed free choice as well as free expression, Dinkins said. The pill was not for Frenchwomen alone, he declared to PPFA. "In truth, the right to choose belongs to women everywhere."

Elections in 1990 suggested growing support for abortion across the country. In Nevada and Oregon, pro-choice measures triumphed. All 1990 gubernatorial candidates in California advocated a pilot program for RU-486.

Sakiz's mail included a letter from seventy congressmen and -women urging Roussel-Uclaf to seek FDA approval for RU-486.

"As elected United States officials," they wrote, "we are greatly concerned that your company's revolutionary new drug, RU-486, may not become available to American women in the near future owing to a variety of real and perceived problems in the current political climate for contraception and abortion. . . . We want to assure you that we are willing to fight to remove, through legislation, policy or regulatory obstacles to medical progress that are motivated by political rather than scientific concerns."

Unquestionably, the tide was rising. Lawrence Tribe of Harvard discussed the pill in *Abortion: Clash of Absolutes* and concluded: "The wide availability of RU-486 could bring truly revolutionary results." Like the AMA, he warned that it had to be tested in America and made legal. "Considering the ease of travel to Europe, a black market in the drug is almost certain. If President Bush's War on Drugs is an uphill battle, if Prohibition was unwinnable, a ban on RU-486 will be a lost cause." This statement is probably exaggerated but it rightly suggests the absurdity of impermeable barriers among our free societies.

One piece of news convinced me that our restive molecule had finally penetrated irreversibly into the rough-and-tumble of American reality: Harvard Business School had begun using the launch of RU-486 as a students' case study.

With all its backing, some proponents urge, RU-486 may find some other legal way into the United States. It might be licensed by one state's authorities and produced there, for example, to give it exposure in at least one place. FDA jurisdiction does not extend to a drug manufactured in one state if it is not transported across state lines.

FDA approval could be sought for RU-486 to treat specific diseases rather than as an abortifacient. As Tribe notes, using licensed drugs for something other than their specified purpose is not against any law; the first birth control pills were sold for menstrual disorders. Many gynecologists prescribe high doses of an oral contraceptive as a "morning-after" pill to stop implantation within three days of intercourse.

My view is that these are the wrong ways. When RU-486 is

made available in America, it should not come in the back door. It should be federally approved for what it is and readily available, administered with the controls and supervision that have worked well in France.

There are a number of possibilities. After successful clinical trials in the United States, the mood might change enough for Hoechst to relent. Roussel-Uclaf could then be free to apply to the FDA and bring its product to America, flags flying. Short of that, a Roussel subsidiary might acquire the rights from its parent corporation and join forces with other partners.

If major companies are hesitant to develop fertility control products, some smaller ones see an opportunity. GynoPharma Inc., a small Somerville, New Jersey, company with the courage to continue marketing an IUD, is among those that have volunteered to handle RU-486.

Roderick L. Mackenzie, chairman of GynoPharma and a veteran in the field, agrees that large companies with diversified products have a lot at risk. But those specializing in reliable gynecological drugs have a large potential. "There is a billion-dollar-a-year business in contraceptives," he said. "If you put aside the Dalkon Shield as an aberration, only twelve lawsuits have been lost in thirty years."

A possible answer is a new single-product company. A carefully designed corporate structure could limit the liability, discouraging nuisance lawsuits and offering no other product to be boycotted. Venture capital could offset the early costs. Private entrepreneurs have offered at least $100 million to allow a jointly owned company to apply to the FDA and begin production. They are convinced that the success in France will repeat itself. Once on the market, with a growing number of firsthand accounts of women able to compare RU-486 with surgical methods, opposition will melt away. As research broadens the range of RU-486, investments may pay off handsomely.

A network of family planning clinics already exists across the country. With the American Medical Association and clinical research centers of medical schools behind RU-486, there would be no shortage of medical personnel.

Until recently, an obstacle in the United States was the lack of a suitable prostaglandin. Roussel policy forbade export to any country where prostaglandins were not readily available. Neither of the compounds used with RU-486 in Europe has been licensed by the FDA. But there is a synthetic prostaglandin, carboprost, sold by Upjohn to control bleeding after childbirth. And now, the misoprostol we have been testing in France is made and sold in America by Searle. The obstacle has been potentially overcome. In the future, the availability and convenience of misoprostol may become crucial if RU-486 is offered under more private conditions than in abortion clinics.

The Lasker award was a major step for our controversial molecule, and it was an immense joy to me. Biology and medicine have produced so many discoveries that no researcher can remain unmoved by recognition from distinguished peers.

The controversy over RU-486 might have worked against me. My award could have brought abuse upon the prestigious Lasker Foundation, and a less responsible body might have sought to avoid the storm. Instead, it demonstrated courage on the part of scientists who nominated me and made me all the prouder to be among them.

Right-to-life zealots declared themselves outraged, but the broad current of humanist science overwhelmed them. At the ceremony, I was thrilled at the presence of people whose work I had long admired. Mary Lasker was there, moving stiffly with age, watching us with her blazing blue eyes. Each of us knew how much medical science owed to her support. Dr. Michael DeBakey, chairman of the jury and one of the world's most honored surgeons, explained that the award is given for quality of work, and it was scientists themselves who made their judgment.

I was informed in advance, but in strict confidence, and could not alert those whom I wanted most to attend, my children and my closest collaborators. I was afraid their pride might overcome their discretion. Only a few days before the ceremony, I told Philippe Lazar, director general of INSERM. With an enthusiasm I won't forget, he quickly caught a plane for New York.

Sometimes I reflect on the prize, trying to better understand where I came from and where I am headed. A lot of others deserved the award, and I knew that defending RU-486 was a factor in the jury decision. My activity was honored because the people who best understood its broad consequences believed that it should be put to work as quickly and widely as possible.

Other distinctions followed. In 1990, Lieberman rang me from New York. "Are you sitting down?" he asked; he knew that I seldom did in my office. He told me I had been elected to the U.S. National Academy of Sciences as a foreign associate. My old friend was as happy for me as I was for myself. I also received the Golden Plate of the American Academy of Achievement, again raising the visibility of RU-486.

Time after time, I repeated my position to American audiences. Abortion is distasteful, but it is an essential recourse. I respect the conscience of those who are against it. Certainly it should not be pushed on anyone who has not decided clearly that she should not, or cannot, complete her pregnancy. But a woman's rights are defined by law. Denying access to a medical means of abortion falls into that category of immorality which the antiabortionists define with such authority.

American women want RU-486 and, sooner rather than later, will bring it to the United States. Researchers will improve on it, synthesize other forms and find other uses in reproductive control. It may end up contributing substantially in fighting several severe illnesses. Or maybe it will do only what we have found it does so well.

As a scientist, I have learned how logical conclusions follow a specific observation. Any doubts that accompanied RU-486 when it first appeared have since been dispelled. False beliefs about the pill have been adjusted to reality. In America, as elsewhere, scientists have embraced it. Just as the obstacles to my visa suddenly dropped away in 1961, I'm convinced the obstacles to RU-486 will be overcome. Politics will give way to science. Maybe because science ultimately offers a real piece of truth.

Chapter Seven

ON A
PLANET APPROACHING
SIX BILLION

IN WEALTHY COUNTRIES like the United States and France, RU-486 is a medical option for safe abortion, sparing women the trauma of surgery. In other parts of the world, it can be the difference between life and death. Whether we like it or not, abortion is a growing trend in most developing countries. Every day, forty thousand children die hungry. Many poor mothers are determined not to produce more.

For all the success of family planning programs, the failure rate of contraceptive use is alarming in developing countries. Women badly need the backup methods of effective contragestion and safe abortion. RU-486 has a vital role to play.

Under Third World conditions, RU-486 can be a safer, more practical, better accepted, and less expensive means to interrupt pregnancy than suction or curettage, and it is clearly an improvement over currently practiced folk methods. It has yet a broader role in countries where contraception is scarcely utilized: helping governments to dampen a population explosion which threatens to outstrip the world's resources.

Scientists are best out of the polemic over whether rich countries ought to seek to limit population in poor countries. But medicine must offer options. As emotive beings, scientists cannot ignore the evidence such as I saw on the Calcutta bridge twenty years ago. Parents have the right to choose a large family. They also have the right to choose a smaller one.

A social transition long since experienced in industrialized countries is now being felt in the Third World. Once rural parents needed children to work the fields, and large families were a sign of wealth. Now, many parents want their children to be educated and well adjusted—and fewer in number.

Leaders are realizing that contraception is not enough, and abortion will be with us for a long time. The laws which once banned it in much of the Third World are changing. Anyone who doubts that legality of abortion has little bearing on its incidence has only to look at Nicolae Ceauşescu's Romania.

Ceauşescu wanted more Romanians at any cost. He not only forbade contraceptives but also made abortion punishable by death. His informers kept a sharp eye out for lawbreakers. The birth rate surged up only briefly. Within a few years, it was lower than ever. Instead of more babies, Ceauşescu brought on the highest rate of dead mothers in Europe.

Romania taught chilling lessons we cannot forget. A woman forced to bear a child is seldom a good mother. After Ceauşescu's fall, the world saw sickening scenes of orphanages where unwanted children lived like caged animals. Even more, Romania showed with brutal clarity what we know from everywhere else in the world: women who want to end their pregnancies will find a way.

Laws cannot stop abortion; they only make it more dangerous. One of the first decrees by the insurgents who deposed Ceauşescu was to legalize abortion. In the following six months, January to July of 1990, the mortality rate from abortions was half that for the same period of 1989.

Over the past twenty years, thirty-six countries have relaxed their abortion laws. More than 2 billion people live in countries which theoretically allow a woman free choice. No other social change has swept the world with such speed. Now the greater problem is not legality but rather guaranteeing a woman's rights and assuring her access to safe methods.

Poor countries can satisfy only a fraction of the demand for early terminations. Too long a wait can mean carrying a pregnancy to term. Often, a woman's only alternative is makeshift medicine which might kill her.

In India, progressive leaders have worried about population problems for decades. Family planners are active, and abortion is legal. But each year, of the 7 million known abortions in India, 6 million take place outside of proper medical facilities. There are not enough surgeons to go around. Eighty percent of Indian women live in the countryside, and all but 7 percent of the doctors live in the cities. Mother Teresa actively dedicates herself to assisting the victims of misery, squalor, disease, and death. Wouldn't it be more appropriate to prevent suffering, instead of accepting it because of religious precepts?

This is no moral or political abstraction; it is a question of survival. Perhaps as many as a million women die each year from causes related to childbearing, including 200,000 from abortion. The rest are victims of pregnancy in desperate circumstances. It is dangerous nonsense to blame abortion for taking unborn lives in countries where unwanted newcomers cause such suffering to those already born. One in five infant deaths could be avoided if mothers spaced their pregnancies at least two years apart.

What I saw in Calcutta is magnified today in almost any city of the Third World. In Nairobi, children abandoned on the street grow up in gangs. Boys filch wallets as soon as they can run, and some start killing in their teens. Girls resort to prostitution before they are ten. And Nairobi is not the worst.

Beyond the broad numbers, Jodi Jacobson offers a close-up look at these problems in a booklet titled *The Global Politics of Abortion*, published by the Worldwatch Institute. Among other cases, she focuses on Zambia, which has one of Africa's most liberal abortion laws.

Abortions are legal through the twelfth week in Zambia, but most are performed outside the period of time permitted by the law. Some women do not know the proper procedures to follow. Many more of them do but cannot get through the maze.

Only the University Teaching Hospital (UTH) can perform abortions, after one specialist and two other physicians sign a form listing a woman's previous births and pregnancies. The doctors must agree on one of three grounds: a medical condition of the woman or of the fetus, or a nonmedical reason which justifies termination. In 1990, only three Zambian specialists were qualified to sign, and one of them lived in Kenya.

Quoted in the booklet, Renée Holt, a nurse and lawyer who studies abortion trends, surveys the situation:

"Obstetricians and gynecologists at UTH did not have enough operating time to perform all the abortions requested. They were turning away half of the requests each day, and these were returning to UTH as incomplete or septic (infected) abortions, which then demanded their time (to save the woman's life), setting up a vicious cycle."

These are discouraging odds in any circumstance. In Zambia, they amount to a nightmare for a worried woman who needs to end her pregnancy. Nothing is easy in Zambian hospitals, where patients must bring their own sheets and soap. For an abortion, the process works like this:

A woman is first screened at the hospital, where many are rejected. If accepted, she is given an appointment which, if she is lucky, is within the time limit for a legal operation. If the doctor she sees opposes abortion, she may be given another appointment at an outpatient clinic. A doctor who agrees to an abortion must get other approvals before giving her a booking date. She must then find her own anesthetic and report for her operation. Often, the caseload is too heavy, and she has to return—if it is not too late.

A typical night at UTH is described in the booklet by Mary Ann Castle, another family planning specialist:

"Ten women were lying, sitting and leaning on nine beds in three rooms . . . five others were sprawled on the concrete floors of the hallway connecting their rooms. A few more were lying or seated on the floor outside the entrance to the Gynecology Admissions Ward. . . . Although the temperature was warm, the dark concrete environment and the condition of the women required blankets or covers. There were none. Many of these women came to the hospital for medical treatment of incomplete, induced abortion. . . . Most wait twelve hours for treatment from a physician. . . . The nurses are often alone with women who are aborting on the floors or on their way to the single toilet at the end of the long hall. 'All we can do is clean up.' Each day three out of ten illegally induced abortion patients complete their abortions on the concrete floor with no medical

care. Nurses are not permitted to give medications or analgesics
without a doctor's prescription.

"According to the nurse in charge, the 'average' woman
ends up overnight on the floor. She receives no food or water
because of the anticipated curettage procedure. [Consequently]
many women are dehydrated . . . increasing the need for intra-
venous fluids once treatment begins. . . . Many are in need of
transfusions by the time they are taken into the operating room.
Some refuse because of fear of HIV infection. Most who need
blood usually do not receive any because of shortages."

These are the lucky ones, among the tiny fraction of women
who receive health care after a bad abortion endangers their life.
Throughout the Third World, the risk over a lifetime of maternal
death is 80 to 600 times higher than in the industrial countries.

No one knows the real numbers. World Health Organization
figures show that at least half a million women die of causes
related to pregnancy each year. We have seen that many of these
are the result of abortions performed with sharp metal, sticks, or
poisons. But studies in individual countries suggest that mortality is far higher. And for every woman who dies, another thirty or
more suffer serious health problems which may last their whole
lives.

Many women resort to dangerous alternatives because they
cannot afford a surgical abortion. In Mexico, for example, women
can find doctors in urban areas, but the rate ranges from $215 to
$665 in an economy where the minimum wage is $103 a month.

Almost all of this suffering can be prevented. The most
effective way, and probably the least expensive way, is with
RU-486.

The bottleneck elsewhere is the lack of surgeons and hospital space. RU-486 can be administered by paramedics in outpatient clinics. In less than 5 percent of the cases, expulsion is
not complete and surgery is needed. The incomplete expulsion
may cause bleeding, which requires a woman to be near medical
assistance. But the danger is no greater than with vacuum aspiration. And it is slight compared with the damage now caused by
unskilled practitioners using other methods.

Far from being too sophisticated for poor countries, as some argue, RU-486 is a much simpler method than surgery. Among many cultures and societies, it is less likely to frighten hesitant women, who would see it as a process closer to nature than surgical means. Taken at an early stage, RU-486 is much less likely to leave fetal tissue than is a poorly performed surgical abortion. This reduces the chance of secondary infection or bleeding.

Progress in the use of prostaglandins will limit the procedure to only a single visit for an abortion, with one follow-up examination after expulsion. If a woman fails to return after taking RU-486 because no expulsion occurred, the result may be that she will have the baby she sought to prevent. Nothing has suggested potential damage to a baby born after treatment with RU-486.

An antiprogesterone works on the uterine wall, not on the embryo. It is quickly passed out of the body. At the stage it is administered, the fetal organs are not developed enough to suffer damage. This cannot be clinically tested on women, but in three cases in England and two in France, in which the women failed to abort after RU-486, did not receive the prostaglandin, and changing their minds, decided against vacuum aspiration, the babies were normal.

Animal trials are reassuring. Embryo damage was found in rabbits that failed to abort after being given purposely insufficient doses of RU-486; some heads were deformed by uterine contractions. But this is a mechanical, not a biochemical, function. Rabbits are the only mammals with such an active uterus. In tests with rats, monkeys, and other species, the result has been healthy births.

Even in developing countries with rudimentary health care, specialized clinics can offer safe administration of RU-486. The term "developing" applies to nations, not individuals. Poor doctors, it need hardly be pointed out, can be as competent as rich ones.

There will always be some risk. Pregnancy is a risk. Life is a risk. The point is that the danger is slight, a tiny fraction of that faced in most countries by women seeking abortion under present circumstances.

It is important not to exaggerate the difficulties. Opponents of RU-486, seeking to keep it out of developed countries, say it is too easy, that it encourages women to have abortions. When they want to block its use in developing countries, they say it is too difficult, that health systems cannot handle it. Neither extreme reflects reality.

RU-486's strongest advocates in the Third World are the specialists who have seen it work. Ethical and emotional judgments are made at a personal level, but medical questions are not for laymen to decide. Clinical physicians and scientific researchers who have performed trials with RU-486 in developing countries are virtually unanimous on its promise.

Dr. Banoo Coyagi, director of K.E.M. Hospital in India's Maharashtra state, found RU-486 to be more culturally acceptable than surgical abortion and easily administered in outpatient clinics. "This is of immense use in the developing world," she wrote in *People*, the magazine of the International Planned Parenthood Federation. "The scope is unlimited."

When Britain's Birth Control Trust met in late 1989, one speaker was José Barzelatto, a Chilean endocrinologist who, succeeding Alex Kessler, had headed the WHO program on human reproduction until June 1989. He had supervised doctors in thirteen countries who tested the pill on three thousand women. Later, he joined the Ford Foundation as senior adviser on population and reproductive health.

Barzelatto said that "limited trained manpower and poor quality of services" in many countries were precisely why RU-486 could be so valuable. The pill could not only ensure more safe abortions than are now possible, he said, but also simplify procedures for women seeking help. "It is hoped that as the availability of the method becomes widely known, the percentage of women consulting early would increase," he said.

In Bangladesh, Barzelatto explained, many women seeking menstrual regulation by vacuum aspiration are rejected because they come too late. But a significant percentage of them have to

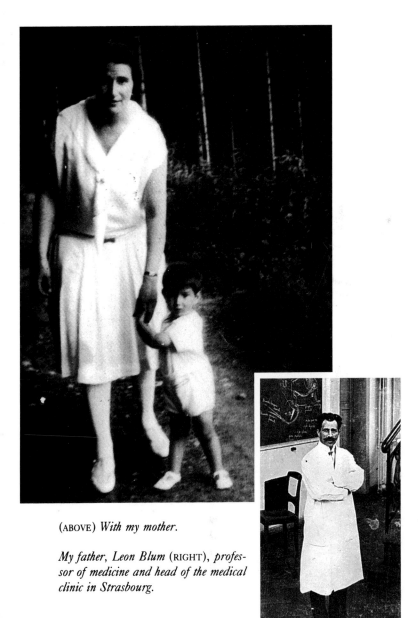

(ABOVE) *With my mother.*

My father, Leon Blum (RIGHT), *professor of medicine and head of the medical clinic in Strasbourg.*

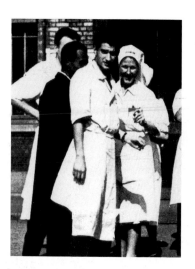

(RIGHT) *In 1948, as a medical student at the Hospital Bichat, where I performed my first surgical abortions.*

(BELOW) *At the Faculty of Medicine in Paris during the sixties.*

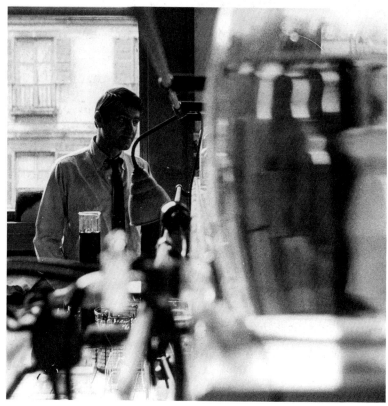

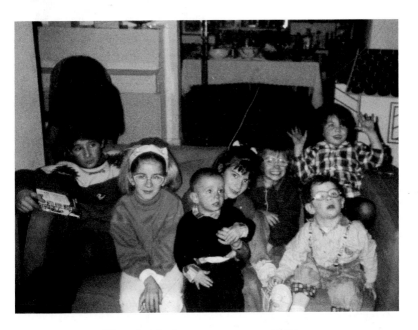

Three decades later, my seven grandchildren.

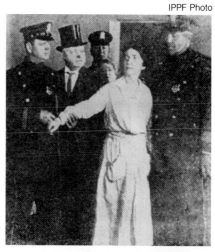

(RIGHT) *Margaret Sanger, arrested in 1916. Sanger was a
pioneer in the birth control movement, and from her base in
Brooklyn established clinics
around the world.*

(BELOW) *Pro-choicers march on
Washington, D.C., November
12, 1989.*

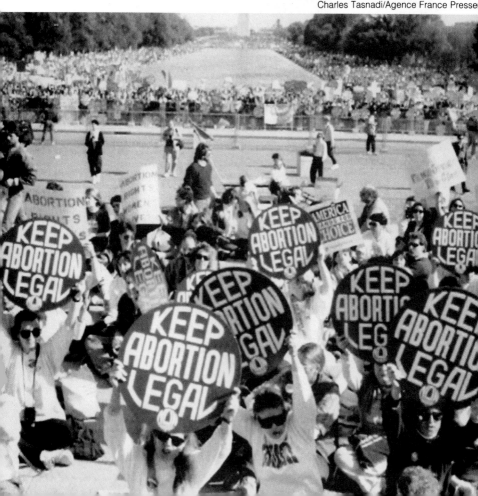

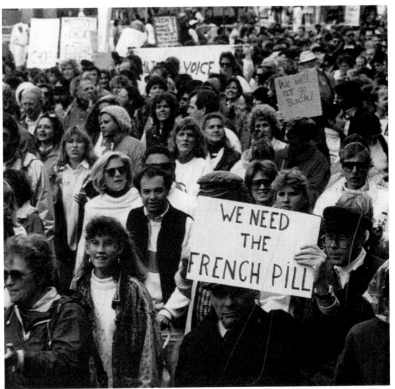

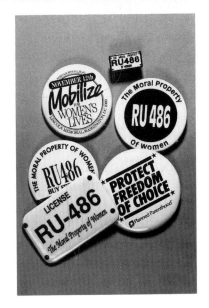

(ABOVE) *The push for RU-486 was already on during the 1989 Washington pro-choice rally.*

(RIGHT) *An assortment of badges in favor of bringing RU-486 into America.*

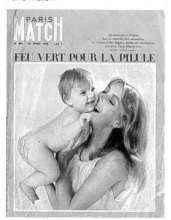

The contraceptive pill is legalized in France in 1966.

(BELOW) *Gregory Pincus invited me to speak at the Lau-
rentian Hormone Conference
in 1965. He (on the left) and
I pause between sessions for a
breath of fresh air.*

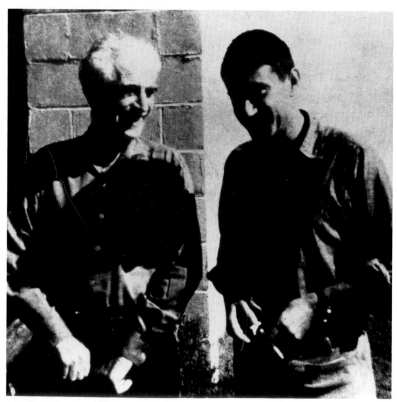

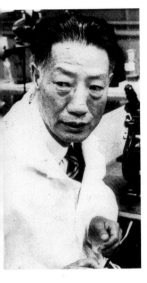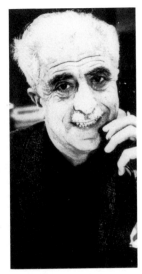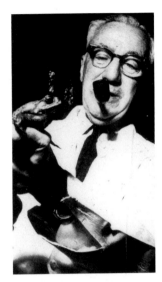

(ABOVE) *The pioneers of oral contraception: From the left, M. C. Chang, Gregory Pincus, and John Rock.*

(RIGHT) *The words of the eminent scientist Carl Djerassi in* The Politics of Contraception, *1979.*

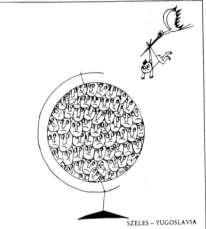

SZELES – YUGOSLAVIA

We act as if we had unlimited time and as if we lived in splendid isolation in a separate world. The price for our myopic perception of global population problems will be a high one which the next generation will have to pay.

CARL DJERASSI

Szeles/Yougoslavy/Rothco in C. Djerassi

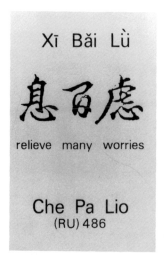

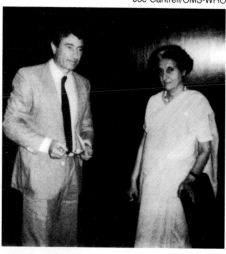

Xī Bǎi Lǜ

息百慮

relieve many worries

Che Pa Lio
(RU) 486

*The Chinese translitera-
tion of "RU-486" con-
verts to a reassuring
phrase.*

(ABOVE) *With Indira
Gandhi in 1983. She
had hoped to see RU-486
introduced into India as
an additional choice for
women.*

(LEFT) *In Thai villages,
abortion is still practiced
by massage.*

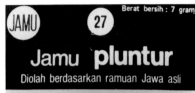

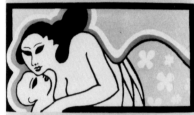

In Indonesia, where abortion is illegal, Jamu, a drug based on plant extracts, is sold without prescription in the markets. Although it is used for abortions, the label calls it "a menstrual regulator" and specifies that it should not be taken in case of pregnancy.

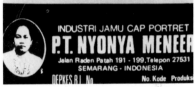

(BELOW) *In Sudan in 1988. Dinka children die of malnutrition, victims of an imbalance between the population and food supply.*

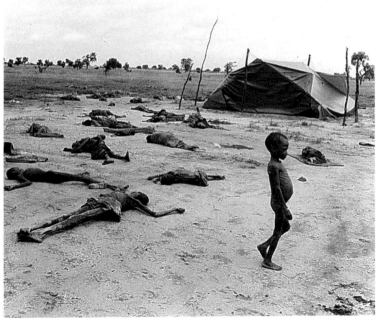

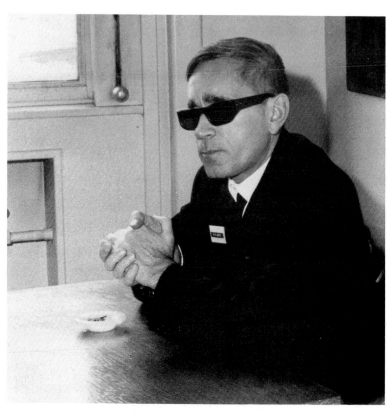

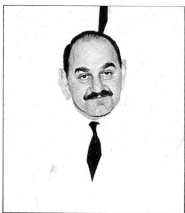

My first boss, the biochemist Max-Fernand Jayle (ABOVE), professor at the Faculty of Medicine in Paris.

(LEFT) My American friend and mentor, the biochemist Seymour Lieberman, during his tenure as professor at the Columbia University School of Medicine.

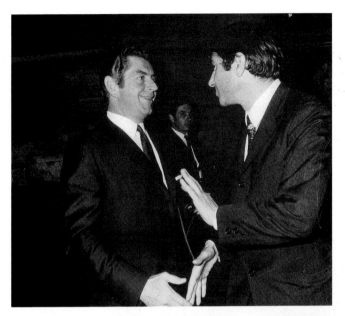

With Jean-Claude Roussel (ABOVE, *on the left*), *former president of Roussel-Uclaf. He was killed in a helicopter accident in 1972.*

(RIGHT) *With Doctor Edouard Sakiz* (*on the right*), *the current president of Roussel-Uclaf.*

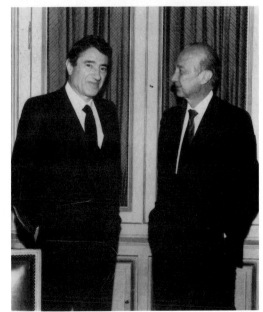

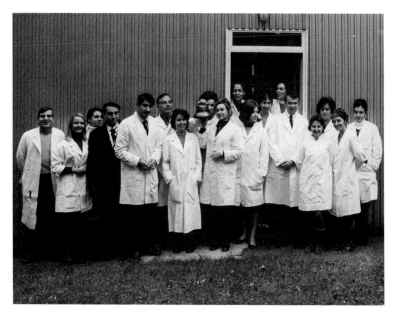

The workers of INSERM research unit U-33 in 1969. We are standing in front of our barracks, which served as a laboratory until 1970.

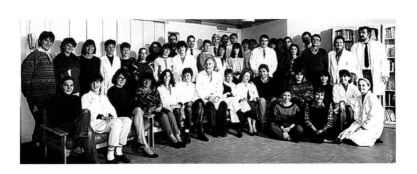

The workers of U-33 in 1990.

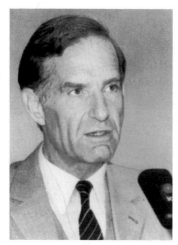

(LEFT) *Wolfgang Hilger, the president of Hoechst, the German parent company of Roussel-Uclaf.*

(BELOW) *Dr. Sakiz's private home in Paris has been the target of pro-lifers.*

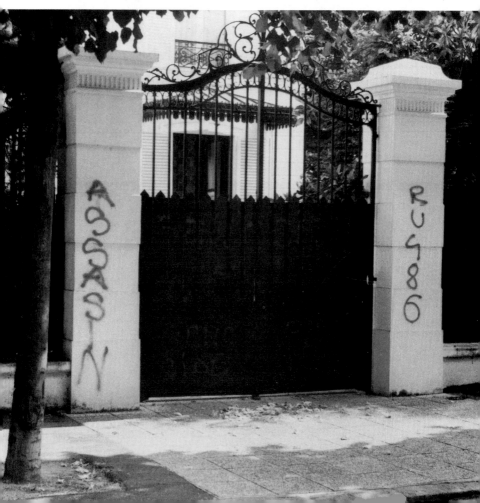

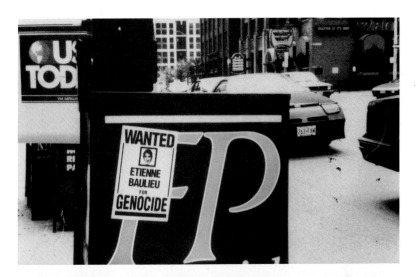

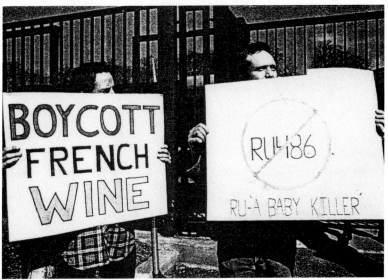

When I gave a talk on RU-486 in Toronto in May 1991, these wanted posters (TOP) *cropped up on the streets of the city.*

(ABOVE) *Anti–RU-486 demonstrators in Washington, D.C.*

S. Lindenberg and J. Falck-Larsen, University of Copenhagen;
S. J. Kimber, University of Manchester; and L. Hamberger,
University of Göteborg

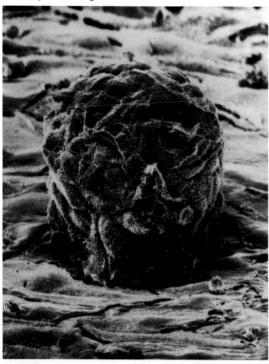

(LEFT) *A fertilized human egg at implantation, the stage at which the egg attaches itself to the wall of the uterus. This unique photograph of the blastocyst attaching to human endometrial cells in culture was taken by a scanning electron microscope.*

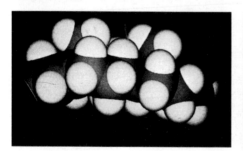

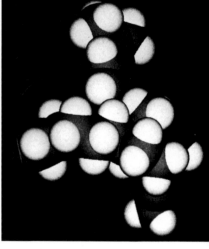

Atomic model of progesterone (LEFT) and RU-486 (RIGHT). The actual length of the molecules is about one-millionth the size of the implanting egg.

wait because they are too early for best results with aspiration. This confuses women about when is the best time to try to get attention from hard-pressed health services. RU-486 would permit a campaign for early care and ease the overload on clinics.

Barzelatto noted that statistics in the Third World seldom reflect an accurate measure of the quality of care. The number of cases requiring a second aspiration or other treatment are underreported. Infection is rife because disposable instruments are used again and again, and sterilization procedures are often inadequate. "The specter of AIDS knocking at the door of Southeast Asia increases this concern, and a medical method of abortion could decrease such complications," he said.

Barzelatto added an important proviso: "Progress must be cautious and accompanied by clear comparative studies so that each country can determine where it is a viable and useful option for them." But he concluded with a ringing endorsement, based on Claude Evin's assertion that RU-486 was the moral property of women.

"Apart from the strictly medical considerations," he said, "is it not a glaring injustice that the most deprived women cannot share the benefits of scientific advances that are helping their more privileged sisters in France to go through the always difficult process of having an abortion by means of a noninvasive procedure with less intrusion into their privacy?"

Each woman's well-being is part of the larger question of demographics. By focusing on dramatic problems such as AIDS, we tend to ignore crises of greater magnitude. Each year in the 1990s, the women who die from botched abortions will outnumber all the people who have died so far from AIDS, but it is AIDS that rivets world attention. During the 1990s, between 5 and 10 million people are expected to die from AIDS. That is the amount of one month's increase in the world population.

If we can help women control the size of their families, we can alleviate the global problems of hunger and overpopulation. By now we have so frequently heard frightening numbers from Africa, Asia, and Latin America that we are inoculated to the shock they once caused. But the numbers grow by the week, and to the people who live with them, they are as real as death.

In 1984, after viewing tragic news film, the world rallied to help Ethiopia. The same famine returns each year, but few of us are watching any longer. At the end of 1990, the U.N. World Food Program estimated that sub-Saharan Africa's food needs for 1991 would exceed those of 1984, when we vowed to abolish hunger in Africa.

On that desperate continent, 80 percent of the food is grown and marketed by women. Esther Ocloo, a Ghanaian entrepreneur and cofounder of Women's World Banking, made the point when she won the Hunger Project's 1990 Africa Prize: "I can assure you that if the right environment and incentives were created for women farmers, and the problems facing them now addressed, the sustainable end of hunger would be a reality." That environment, she said, requires freedom from the strain of unwanted childbearing.

Demographics are changing fast. In the past, women died before their men, if not victims of childbirth, then weakened by rearing large families. Now, on average, women in wealthy countries outlive men by eight years. In most of the Third World, these numbers do not apply. Often women die long before their time, leaving behind large families their husbands cannot feed.

When I joined the WHO committee on human reproduction in the mid-1960s, there were 3.5 billion people in the world, and the number increased by 70 million a year. Today, there are 5.3 billion people, and the annual increase is 90 million. That is, each year the world's population goes up by the equivalent of the population of Mexico. But, at the present rate, Mexicans alone will number 600 million by 2050, more than twice the population of the United States today.

A child born today can expect to live in a world with twice the present population before he is forty.

Bangladesh is making progress in birth control, but its population is expected to double before it may stabilize. That will mean a population the size of the United States and in a country no bigger than Wisconsin and with few resources. India now has 830 million people, and its yearly increase equals the population of Holland.

In percentage terms, the increase in world population has dropped slightly, from 2 percent to 1.8 percent. And yet every four days there are 1 million more births than deaths. If a bomb equal to that dropped on Hiroshima had fallen every day since August 6, 1945, world population would still be on the rise.

And yet, even modest efforts can make an impact. Jessica Mathews of the World Resources Institute made a simple calculation, based on a progression of threes: "A young woman today who bears 3 children instead of the 6 her mother may have borne will have 27 great-grandchildren instead of 216."

Back in 1965, the late Sir Dugald Baird, David Baird's father, then Regius Professor of Obstetrics and Gynecology at the University of Aberdeen, Scotland, wrote a landmark paper entitled "The Fifth Freedom." He listed the four basic rights described in the 1940s by President Franklin D. Roosevelt: freedom of speech and worship, freedom from want and fear. To that, Sir Dugald added "freedom from the tyranny of excessive fertility."

In 1990, the British journal *Lancet* recalled Sir Dugald's bold assertion. "The challenge of the next twenty-five years is to bring global population close to stabilization," *Lancet* commented. "In order to achieve the low (or even median) population projection for the twenty-first century, there must be universal availability of family planning services by the year 2000 and a doubling of the number of couples using modern methods of contraception in the decades of the '90s. Realistic policies are required in breastfeeding, contraceptive distribution, voluntary surgical contraception, abortion, management and the need for more human and financial resources."

Lancet concluded: "If there were no unintended pregnancies in the world, human population would stabilize at under 8 billion. If there is no further improvement in family planning, it could drift to 14 billion. The choice is an important one."

It could hardly be more important. The difference between

the two *Lancet* projections is 6 billion people within a few generations, more than today's total population.

In 1991, United Nations experts revised their population projections, shifting them sharply upward. According to new estimates, world population is likely to reach 6.4 billion people by the year 2001, rising to 10 billion before 2050.

These catastrophic numbers are worsened by urbanization. By 2010, half the people on earth will live in large cities, already suffering from appalling slums, crime, pollution, and disease. In 1950, there were ten cities of more than 5 million inhabitants. Now there are thirty-five; six of them surpass 15 million inhabitants. In many of them, growing squalor threatens epidemics and famine. The poorest continent, Africa, will have three times the population of North America by the year 2025.

If morality is an issue in family planning, morality demands action. It is not enough to moralize in theory and hold fast to fixed ideas. Politics have no place here.

The Reagan administration set back progress critically in 1984 with its Mexico City Policy on foreign aid. American funds were denied to any agency or program that dealt with abortion, even if the abortion component was supported only by non-U.S. funding. The impact was devastating. International agencies abandoned important work. Six years later, American abortion rights activists lost a court case to change the policy. In Bangladesh, some government hospitals refused to assist women who had attempted their own abortions, endangering their lives, for fear of losing American aid.

However much politicians and moralists try to draw a distinction, abortion remains a key component of family planning. In Latin America, about a quarter of fertility control is by induced abortion. As Jodi Jacobson concluded, "Contraceptives reduce, but do not eliminate, the need for abortion as a backup to their own failure."

Increasingly, there will be a role for contragestion, the middle ground between classical contraception and abortion. RU-486 will be crucial to this, offering a backup method to contraceptives.

The *Lancet* editorial was based on an article by Malcolm Potts and Allan Rosenfield, "The Fifth Freedom Revisited." Potts is a physician who works extensively in family planning, and Rosenfield is dean of the Columbia University School of Public Health. Among other points, the authors noted: "All those who are genuinely disturbed by the tens of millions of abortions that take place each year must work together to help bring about a significant reduction in that number by advocating a marked increase in investment in family planning services and in support of contraceptive research. Without such a change, it is possible that more legal and illegal abortions will be induced in the 1990s than in any previous decade of human history. Whatever happens with funding, there is no doubt that universal access to safe abortion could save the lives of millions of women in the 1990s."

Addressing these problems does require a lot of money, on balance. By United Nations estimates, the funds required for effective birth control programs in the Third World amount to one dollar per year for every citizen living in industrialized nations.

RU-486's place in the Third World remains to be defined. There are substantial barriers to be overcome.

Roussel-Uclaf's current export policy virtually excludes developing countries from directly buying the compound or making it under license. Only industrialized countries with closely monitored pharmacy distribution and well-run modern clinics are under consideration.

By contrast, the World Health Organization can assure a supply to any qualifying country which officially requests the drug. WHO's intervention on behalf of China in 1990 was an important precedent. But the U.N. agency's eagerness to distribute RU-486 remains to be tested. It is not clear to what degree the U.S. government discourages WHO from supporting RU-486, and U.N. officials privately admit reluctance to invite the wrath of conservative American authorities.

Some specialists worry that RU-486 could represent a medical risk in rural areas where women cannot easily return to a clinic for follow-up. This concern comes from lack of experience with the pill; its risk is less than that of surgical methods. But skeptical professionals must be convinced.

In reality, RU-486 by itself does not carry a risk; it can only improve the present catastrophic situation regarding pregnancy in the developing world. The true problem is that the very state of pregnancy is and will remain a risk to a woman's health whether or not it is wanted. Thus, complications may be falsely but loudly attributed to RU-486, perpetuating the negative rumors.

The Program for Appropriate Technology in Health (PATH), a nonprofit, nongovernmental group based in Seattle, received a private grant to design model programs for introducing RU-486 into the Third World. Its experts are looking into concerns expressed over possible risk to rural patients.

Other barriers are broader, reflecting general attitudes toward fertility control in regions of the Third World.

John and Pat Caldwell, brilliant demographers from Australia, noted that six times as many Asian women as African women practice efficient birth control. Sub-Saharan Africa, they wrote in *Scientific American*, "is not more traditional, primitive, or backward; it is simply very different, and the differences have profound implications."

Social, cultural, and economic reasons push African men toward large families, often with many wives, and African women continue to pursue motherhood. But, the Caldwells wrote, there are signs of change. At the World Population Conference in Bucharest in 1974, Africans were deeply suspicious of family planning programs. Only Kenya and Ghana took part. Ten years later, in Mexico City, almost all African governments supported the idea. Nigeria, with one fourth of the continent's population, is rigorously trying to limit families to four children.

In Latin America, the Catholic Church retains much of its traditional influence. Abortion is illegal in many places, if common, and methods to encourage it are not likely to take hold any time soon. However, movement within the Church offers some grounds for optimism. Religious doctrine is one thing, but a growing number of priests see the conflict between the Church's good work and the pain that Vatican stringency can cause. Like most of us, they have looked into the eyes of too many poor, hungry children. The growing influence of Protestant churches in Latin America is also liberalizing the general climate. Since 1931, for instance, the Federal Council of the Churches of Christ has insisted on a "new morality" based on freedom and knowledge.

In each country, the future of RU-486 depends on national authorities responding to the advice of their medical specialists. For authoritarian governments, a simple decree might be enough to introduce the drug. Among the democracies, the decision might be debated, and good intention may have to work its way through the labyrinth of an entrenched civil service.

Patience is a luxury we cannot afford. When I first spoke with Indira Gandhi of a contraceptive pill twenty years ago, she wanted an Indian pill. In 1983, as prime minister, she volunteered to implement the use of RU-486. Ever since an assassin took her life the following year, the pill's fate in India has remained in suspense. Authorities asked for it, but the paperwork stalled. One of its early advocates, Dr. Vera Hingorani, is pushing hard. Yet it is still available in India only for sporadic clinical trials.

Hesitation must be overcome. The situation, already calamitous, is getting worse. Simple human concern is reason enough to help, but pressing factors in the Third World directly affect richer nations. Resources are unfairly distributed, and the lack of demographic ecology threatens our planet's future. People ravage the land in an ever-widening search for food and fuel. Forests are disappearing, and deserts are advancing. Desperation leads to political upheaval. And as we know too well, turmoil has a way of spilling across national borders.

World population has to be stabilized below 10 billion; the alternative does not bear thinking about. Medical science must be allowed to help. The U.N. Universal Declaration of Human Rights assures "the right of everyone to the enjoyment of the highest obtainable standard of physical and mental health." Everyone, it adds, must "enjoy the benefits of scientific progress and its applications." It does not specify rich or poor.

RU-486 should be put to use along with other tools for maternal health and fertility control as part of broad-based programs to educate women about their new choices. In Africa, as John and Pat Caldwell suggest, comprehensive family planning might be combined with an urgent campaign to stop the spread of AIDS.

We have no time to lose. As the Caldwells said it, "This task is the greatest challenge for international aid in modern times, and posterity will not forgive our generation if we do not meet it."

Chapter Eight

A
DIFFERENT
FUTURE

RU-486, which sprang into the world as the "abortion pill," appears to be what we had hoped it would be from the beginning: a versatile tool in fertility control, but it can also treat serious disease. We are still probing its potential. Whatever comes next, this second-generation pill can help us all shape a different future.

With the publication of our first results, specialists in different fields saw the promise of an antiprogesterone and anticortisone drug. That is a thrilling part of medicine. Each new discovery opens the way to others. A discoverer inadvertently adds pieces to puzzles halfway around the world, just as others' findings had helped him.

My main interest was research into RU-486's potential to help women master their own fertility. For me, the promise of a different future is closely linked to every woman's ability to decide when, and whether, she wants a child.

At the same time, experiments with RU-486 brought spectacular results, as well as vague and unconfirmed hopes, in diverse areas of pathology. An antihormone can act against any corresponding activity. Brief exposure to RU-486 can stop pregnancy. Prolonged use over weeks or months may influence a variety of maladies.

Endometriosis was a likely target. Although the disease affects up to 10 percent of women, it is poorly understood and difficult to treat. It is an excess growth of the uterine lining, which causes pain during menstruation and excessive bleeding, and is often associated with infertility.

Gary Hodgen, at the Jones Foundation laboratories in Virginia, used RU-486 to treat a similar ailment in monkeys. He found an antiestrogen effect, curious since there is no binding with the estrogen receptor. A second result was a drop in LH, the luteinizing hormone, which permits the ovaries to rest. Those combined effects improved the animals' condition.

In San Diego, a brilliant endocrinologist, Samuel Yen, organized studies to apply RU-486. He found encouraging results with women suffering from mild endometriosis, and his work is continuing. He also obtained remarkable regression of uterine fibroids, a condition mostly affecting women of 30 to 40 years of age, and a major indication of hysterectomy.

Meningiomas, tumors in the membrane around the brain, have long challenged doctors. Though benign, they can grow extensively and exert pressure which can be fatal. Some of them are inoperable; they cannot be removed without risking damage to the brain. Meningiomas often contain large amounts of progesterone receptor, and preliminary tests show that RU-486 can sometimes stop their growth.

Cushing's syndrome is produced by an excess of cortisone-related hormones. It is frequently caused by cancer in the adrenal glands or in other organs which send stimuli to the adrenals. High hormone levels can cause hypertension and a tendency to bleed, impeding surgery. Scientists at the National Institutes of Health have found that large doses of RU-486 can counter these cortisone effects so that tumors can be removed. This is a case of the "death pill" saving lives.

The antiglucocorticosteroid effect of RU-486 may be helpful in combating stress disorders, some types of depression, certain cases of high blood pressure, and certain problems of aging. It might also strengthen the body's immune system. Scientists are investigating its impact on diseases ranging from obesity to Alzheimer's.

In the research, ways must be found to counter natural defenses that limit the long-term use of an anticorticosteroid. The body tends to secrete more corticosteroids to balance the activity of RU-486 given orally. However, local use of RU-486 does not bring defenses into play and early clinical results with topical application are exciting.

Applied directly in small doses, RU-486 may hasten the healing of severe burns and wounds. Studies in France are looking into these possibilities. Attempts to treat glaucoma by applying RU-486 directly into the eye are still inconclusive.

The most dramatic possibility is with breast cancers, which kill 43,000 women each year in the United States alone. A number of these cancers have progesterone receptors. In the mid-1980s, my longtime colleague Henri Rochefort showed how RU-486 could inhibit the growth of cancer cells which he cultured at his laboratory in Montpellier.

Roussel-Uclaf accepted for treatment more than thirty women with advanced metastatic breast cancers, especially those who did not respond to tamoxifen, an antiestrogen. In the tests, conducted in France and Holland, about 25 percent of the cases reacted very positively to RU-486. The company agreed to sponsor joint research in France and at the National Cancer Institutes of NIH and Canada.

Despite the pill's controversial role in abortion, Roussel-Uclaf has supported a number of research programs in this and other areas. Long-term use requires careful investigation into possible toxicity and side effects. Medical research is costly, and expense must be weighed against potential gains.

Data already available from the wide use of RU-486 is an advantage. Roussel-Uclaf is able to conduct breast cancer trials directly on women because RU-486 is already safely in use.

RU-486 has an important role in therapeutic abortions. If a woman is ill, or if she is carrying a deformed fetus, doctors may recommend that she terminate her pregnancy. Since progesterone is secreted throughout pregnancy, RU-486 can be effective during the second and third trimesters as well as the first.

Larger amounts of RU-486 are needed in therapeutic applications because the hormone level increases progressively throughout pregnancy. Until now, RU-486 has been used essentially to facilitate second-trimester abortions induced by prostaglandin or curettage. Our first cases were fetuses that had died in about the sixth month and were not expulsed.

RU-486 has been used in patients for whom a rigid cervix prolonged the pregnancy—postterm pregnancy—which is harm-

ful to the child. We have been careful to ensure that this use does
not put the child in danger from the drug. Although the compound is rapidly eliminated, it passes from the mother to the
baby. Experiments on animals in Hodgen's laboratory had suggested that this was no risk. Hodgen's tests, during years of
observation, showed no toxicity or secondary effects on offspring.

A team of French gynecologists reported in *Lancet* early in
1991 on clinical trials with sixty-two women needing induced
labor, half on RU-486 and half on placebo. RU-486 substantially
eased oxytocin-facilitated delivery, and spared some women the
necessity of a cesarean section. Doctors reported no side effects.

The therapeutic use of RU-486 late in delivery is still experimental. No damage has been reported to mothers or fetuses.
But researchers are refining dosages and testing different compounds that might be used with RU-486. It is already a valuable
tool for medical necessity, but I hardly recommend it to speed a
delivery for the parents' or doctors' convenience.

For all its medical value, RU-486's great promise is in preventing
pregnancy in the first place. Beyond what it now does, it may
soon be able to intercept a zygote before implantation, regularly
and reliably, or even prevent ovulation. A woman might use it
occasionally instead of ingesting hormones daily, or living with
diaphragms or IUDs, or resorting to suction if she is late.

The idea certainly is not to replace other methods but rather
to offer a greater choice. If we are to have the enlightened future
Margaret Sanger foresaw half a century ago, women must be free
to control their own bodies. Parents must be free to shape their
families, so that children will be born to mothers prepared to
raise them. A stabilized world population could then sustain itself.

Today, the most common and effective method of birth control
is sterilization. If people must mutilate themselves, decide once
and for all to forgo the chance for procreation, this is a defeat for
us all. Why not address the issue with reversible means?

This method does have a clear advantage. It settles the

question permanently, with no hormonal effect. Vasectomy in the man has nothing to do with castration, which removes the hormone-producing testes. In the woman, tying off the fallopian tubes blocks that primordial race, the pursuit of sperm after the egg. Otherwise, the woman's system functions normally.

Sterilization is favored by parents who have established their families, usually those over thirty-five. But lives can change. Women may bear children up to the age of fifty, and men are fertile far longer.

Besides abstinence, the oldest method of birth control is the condom. It dates back at least to the linen sheath fashioned in 1563 by Gabriele Falloppio, the Italian surgeon who charted the female reproductive tract. Back then, it was to protect against syphilis, and the condom still has the advantage of preventing sexually transmitted disease. Newer barrier forms, such as cervical caps and the diaphragm, share a disadvantage. They must be inserted, defensively and often ostentatiously, before each act of intercourse.

Spermicides fall into a similar category. Though based on a chemical action, they must be physically applied before intercourse. Their additional drawback is a high failure rate.

An intrauterine device offers some of the advantages of sterilization. It is always there. The body functions normally. But the zygote does not implant. The IUD does not prevent sperm from entering the uterus, but reactions of the uterus may help to impede fertilization. Thus the IUD is doubly contragestive.

Despite memories of the Dalkon Shield scandal which still cloud feelings about intrauterine devices, new ones are well designed, effective, and inexpensive over the long run. At the same time, an IUD has its disadvantages. Young women who have not had children cannot use it. A lot of others find it painful or annoying. There is always a slight risk of infection, along with a slightly higher risk of ectopic pregnancy.

Researchers are at work on what might amount to a biological IUD, a vaccination against pregnancy. The only progress yet reported is with a method of neutralizing hCG (human chorionic gonadotropin), the hormone released when an embryo implants, which activates the corpus luteum to secrete more progesterone. Starved of progesterone, the newly implanted embryo would be dislodged. If the method works, it would be comparable with automatically triggering RU-486 at implantation.

Oral contraceptives remain a popular choice; a range of variations work on the principle of Pincus's first-generation pill. The 60 million women who use the pill should be over 99 percent safe from unwanted pregnancy. But women often forget to take the pill, or stop taking it for temporary medical reasons, or simply do not understand that it must be taken for twenty-one days without fail. In some countries, the failure rate is higher than 10 percent.

Doctors agree that the use of oral contraceptives has improved women's health dramatically by sparing them unwanted pregnancies. But some wonder whether it is good to take hormones almost continually. Younger people raise new questions, especially as the old debate lingers over whether the pill adds to the risk of breast cancer. Estrogens are blamed for certain metabolic problems. And some women feel nauseated or bloated on the pill.

"Minipills" of lower doses are popular, but they are less effective. Although minipills are not as apt to systematically block ovulation, the hormones they contain upset the rhythm of the endometrium, so that an embryo does not implant. This principle was behind the "micropills," synthetic progestins without estrogen which were widely used early in the 1970s. Now these have been mostly replaced by implants and injected long-term progestins.

Depo-Provera injections, still banned in the United States, are used by millions of women. But Norplant was approved in America in late 1990. It is a cluster of small tubes implanted in the arm. The tubes can be removed at any time but, once in place, they can be forgotten for years. The drawback is that a continuous supply of progestins can trigger intermittent bleeding.

RU-486 is an effective backup to all contraceptive methods. It has obvious advantages for women who feel they need protection only occasionally. With RU-486, a woman can wait to decide whether she needs birth control. If not, she absorbs no unnecessary hormones and need not bother with mechanical means. If she thinks she risks pregnancy, especially if a period is late, she can take the pill. This amounts to a medical means of menstrual regulation, avoiding the intrusion of vacuum aspiration. It also is known that the failure rate, however small, is slightly higher for aspirations performed prior to seven or eight weeks (it decreases significantly later). This is when RU-486 is particularly efficient.

A healthy young woman who has intercourse around the fifteenth day of her cycle, has on average a one in five, or 20 percent, chance of fertilization, amounting to a risk of two or three pregnancies a year. RU-486 alone taken later, before the end of the cycle, is 80 percent effective in carrying off a fertilized egg. This leaves her with a 4 percent chance of pregnancy, probably less if she takes the misoprostol prostaglandin in addition (trials suggest under 1 percent). If the egg has not been fertilized, she merely advances the end of her cycle without affecting the timing of the next.

However, if there is fertilization but no pregnancy develops, the following ovulation may come later than usual, making the regular use of RU-486 difficult. Work on this option—as a once-a-month menses inducer—is being pursued, testing lower dosages of RU-486 in appropriate association with prostaglandin. In Stockholm, Marc Bygdeman is working on a different once-a-month regimen: low doses of RU-486 just after ovulation to lower the progesterone action in the endometrium and prevent implantation. The problem is to determine when ovulation occurs. Sam Yen and I favor administering a low dose of RU-486 during the entire luteal phase, in order to overcome the difficulty.

We are now trying small doses of RU-486 and misoprostol as a once-a-month method to induce menstruation. If doses are low enough, timing of menstrual cycles may not be affected.

In other trials, Horatio Croxatto, a Chilean specialist, and Tapani Luukkainen in Finland, give RU-486 at the beginning of a cycle to suppress early progesterone action so that no egg is released. A progestin, given later, helps the uterine mucus develop and a second dose of RU-486 can trigger bleeding.

These studies could lead to a new type of estrogen-free oral contraceptive. It would mean long and costly testing, however, resulting in a method that would still require women to take pills for several weeks a month. A question remains whether any company would undertake development. But it is yet another option. There will be others. Will nonprofit family planning organizations be interested in sponsoring research and development in this critical field?

Colleagues at INSERM see me spending hours with journalists and family planning associations and wonder at the time I still devote to the future of RU-486. The people I speak with about RU-486 are just as surprised that I no longer work on fertility control in the laboratory but concentrate on biochemical studies of receptor function and hormones in the central nervous system during aging. Dehydroepiandrosterone sulfate levels decrease with age, and it has been suggested that its administration could slow down the aging process. The substance that launched my research is piquing my interest anew.

I have always been motivated by my scientific curiosity and, at the same time, I want to take part in advancing science to benefit society. These are my two reasons to live. I cannot put one aside to pursue the other.

Ever since I threw rocks at Nazis after school, I have felt a desire to be involved. The personal attacks have hurt. Any scientist would rather be compared with Pasteur than with Hitler. Ironically, the bloody dictators of modern times (Hitler, Stalin, Khomeini, Idi Amin, Ceauşescu) have ferociously opposed the practice of abortion in their respective countries. But in the larger scheme of things, insults mean nothing. The issues for the future do not involve a single product or any one researcher. They are how human societies look at life.

For RU-486, the moral and ethical questions are likely to remain open forever. Emotions surrounding abortion run high. Those of us who respect science, and who champion the woman's choice, can only examine the arguments of the other side and counter them with reason.

* * *

In the debate over abortion, the crucial issue is when a human being begins to exist. No one can settle that question. An energetic minority holds that an individual is given life at the moment of fertilization. But a personal interpretation of God's design does not entitle anyone to deny others a choice which they believe is a basic human right.

It has always been that way in human society. A well-organized, articulate group draws a moral definition and seeks to impose it on a majority. Sometimes the majority embraces the definition. Sometimes they reject it, and the minority cannot muster the power to prevail. Today, the question is whether a moral definition that so deeply affects the life of each individual, and the world at large, can be left to the minority.

Specialists who are qualified to decide when life begins throw up their hands at the task. Scientists of different disciplines have delved deeply into the question. They come up only with explanations, not answers.

In the early 1980s, the British government asked a distinguished panel, chaired by Dame Mary Warnock, to define this crucial issue. The report concluded, "Although the questions of when life or personhood begin appear to be questions of fact susceptible to straightforward answers, we hold that the answers to such questions in fact are complex amalgams of factual and moral judgements."

John D. Biggers, of the Harvard Medical School, is regarded by colleagues as among the world's most qualified experts on early development. In *Human Reproduction*, he warned that disagreement over the word "embryo" tempts policymakers into restrictive decisions on test-tube fertilization, embryo transfer, or contragestives, such as IUDs or RU-486. He argued that any variation of semantics that suggests a distinct demarcation in the definition of "embryo" draws an artificial line in what is actually a seamless process.

He concludes, " 'Embryo' has never been defined on a fundamental basis because the partitioning of prenatal life requires arbitrary decisions that identify transitions in a continuous process called the life cycle. . . . If the moral value of prenatal human life increases as an individual develops, the change in moral value should also form a continuum. Any partitions of this continuum may well be arbitrary."

In the language of scientific papers, he is stressing a point that others make frequently: policymakers and moralists cannot be allowed to distort science to bolster their arguments.

Biggers made his point another way in a chapter of the book *Infertility: A Comprehensive Text*, published in 1989: "We have come through several centuries of fables about generation into an era in which the facts of generation are understood scientifically in terms of the life cycle. All phases of the cycle are living and all members of the human life cycle are genetically unique. Do we now want to adhere to the nonscientific fable that life begins at conception in making ethical decisions?"

Anne McLaren, of the University of London, a leading embryologist, explored the subject in *Proceedings of the Royal Institute*. Her title echoed Biggers's concern: "Where to draw the line." She posed five questions she did not attempt to answer. When does life begin? When does an embryo become human? When does it become a human being? When does it become a unique individual? When does it become conscious?

These, she pointed out, were the wrong questions. "You and I are alive, unborn babies are alive, embryos, fertilized eggs, unfertilized eggs, sperm, and the germ cell that give rise to them—all are alive, and all are human. Human life is a continuum."

After the primitive streak, when the embryo takes on its individual character, it is all but impossible to fix the landmark in development that converts a human life form into a human being. With ultrasound scanning, researchers have noted faint movements at around six weeks, and by fourteen weeks, the movement becomes coordinated. "Quickening," the term used in early legal definition, takes place at sixteen to eighteen weeks, when the movements are strong enough for a mother to detect them. This is an important landmark for the mother, McLaren noted, "but perhaps less so for the fetus."

At about twenty weeks, patterns of total activity begin to appear: body and eye movements, heart rate, and breathing rhythm; by twenty-six weeks, they are organized in distinct phases. Electrical activity in the brain is seen at twenty-two weeks. Between twenty-eight and thirty-two weeks, the neural circuits in the brain are about as advanced as they are at birth. Even at birth, however, electrical brain activity is very immature.

The scientific problem McLaren poses is to define brain function. If it is the distinction between waking and sleep periods, this occurs only in the ninth month of pregnancy. If it is the first electrical impulses in the brain—the reverse definition of brain death—it is weeks earlier.

Viability is a commonly used criterion. Some fetuses as young as twenty-two weeks after fertilization have been kept alive in incubators, but they are unable to suck nourishment or to breathe on their own.

In the end, McLaren wrote, you cannot draw the line. "Any lines that you draw are going to be to some extent arbitrary, and where you finally decide to draw them must depend on the context, the purpose of your decision."

She noted that she had avoided discussing fetal capacity to feel pain or discomfort, the question of consciousness and the intrinsic or potential value of the fetus at different stages. McLaren wrote, "These are issues that involve more than just science. Where you draw the line involves ethical judgments, which I have been careful not to make. But these ethical judgments can and should be based on a correct understanding of what is actually going on at the scientific level."

Helga Kuhse and Peter Singer, of the Center for Human Bioethics at Monash University in Australia, picked up the question where McLaren left it. They discuss the criterion of "sentience," the capacity to feel pleasure or pain, to suffer or to enjoy life. From the evidence assembled, they wrote, "it appears that it is only quite late in its development—possibly in the third trimester of pregnancy—that the brain of the fetus is sufficiently developed for the fetus to be sentient."

Their judgment, like McLaren's, is that all elements of fetal development involve human life. But they go farther. They argue that *any* decision regarding reproduction can be seen as a decision for or against a new human life. It is not just contraception or abortion that precludes new life; even abstinence, with egg and sperm not getting together in the first place, falls into this category.

By logical reasoning, their argument runs, a decision to break a date during those few days of fertility can stop a future life just as decisively as an abortion.

To illustrate the lengths to which moral hair-splitting can go, Kuhse and Singer offer a series of hypothetical situations. In the first, doctors attempting in vitro fertilization have obtained a fertile egg from a woman and some semen from her husband. Just before dropping the semen into the glass dish with the egg, the woman's physician calls to say he has learned that she has a hopeless medical condition and cannot support a pregnancy. The egg could be fertilized and transferred to her womb but would not implant. As a result, the egg and the sperm are separately dumped into the sink.

According to the traditional view, nothing immoral has occurred. But take the second case: Everything happens the same except that the physician's call comes later, after the sperm has fertilized the egg. The couple asks that the egg be disposed of as soon as possible. Now the moral questions start. Is there a human being in the balance?

And there is a third case. The same situation occurs as in the first; sperm and egg go separately down the sink. As fate would have it, the sink is blocked by a surgical dressing. A nurse discovers this and is about to clear it. Suddenly, she has a thought: Perhaps fertilization has occurred. Is she about to commit murder?

Kuhse and Singer come down to the main point of this counting of angels on a pinhead:

"To devote so much time and intellectual energy to the debate of whether eggs, sperm, or zygotes have 'rights' and whether there is a moral difference between destroying those cells, and not bringing them into existence in the first place, may seem almost an obscenity when conducted in a world in which women cannot control their reproductive processes, and in which there are already too many people, and thousands of children are dying each day because their parents can't feed them. Surely, what's important is not whether there is an intrinsic moral difference between abortion and contraception, but rather what role these techniques can play in curbing the population explosion."

The respect and protection we provide individuals from the very start of their potential existence should not be at the expense of identifiable individuals—the members of an existing family, adults and children. It is for each family to decide for itself, with safe, effective measures offered by new techniques. Those who fight against fertility control end up causing even more abortions, and in the worst circumstances.

Organized religions have no clearer answer than science on when a human life begins. The Bible condemns murder but is silent on abortion. Protestants, for the most part, regard it as an unfortunate necessity. Opinions vary among Protestant denominations, but few churchmen regard the early termination of pregnancy as murder. No major Asian faith attempts to name a precise moment when a new person joins the world.

Jewish teachings fix a time, near quickening, when the soul enters the fetus. Until then, the fetus is considered a life form but not a human being, or *nefesh* in Hebrew. Orthodox Jews frown on abortion except to protect the mother's health. Conservative Jews accept "severe anguish" as a sufficient reason. Reform Judaism takes a liberal stand, including the grounds of "freedom of choice."

In a policy paper, Rabbi Aryeh Spero, of the Orthodox Civic Center Synagogue in Manhattan, noted that Jewish tradition dictates that abortions should be done as early as possible, preferably before the fortieth day.

Moslems accept the need for abortion under a number of circumstances. According to the Koran, it becomes the taking of a life only after a process described as "the blowing of the spirit." This is generally believed to occur at the end of the fourth month of pregnancy. I understand that menstrual regulation is not condemned by the Islamic religion.

The Roman Catholic Church, in contrast, holds that fertilization implies the onset of human personhood.

At the height of the controversy over RU-486, Jean-Marie Cardinal Lustiger, the archbishop of Paris, wrote me, challenging my knowledge of Catholic doctrine. "You do not understand that the voluntary interruption of pregnancy is directly contrary to the commandment of God: Thou shalt not kill." No civilized person could disagree with God's commandment. The question is over what is murder.

But I had another view from the Reverend Norman Ford, an Australian priest whose book *When Did I Begin?*, published in 1988, is a classic work in the religious debate. He said he strongly disagreed with the philosophical reading of biology, common but not universal within the Church, that life begins at conception. Father Ford's own view is that an individual is defined after the primitive streak at fourteen days after fertilization. Among contemporary Catholic theologians, he is hardly alone.

Times change. Today's Catholic doctrine has its roots among the Romans, when every conception was the making of another member of an imperiled church. The verb itself, "to conceive," comes from the Latin, *concipere,* "to retain." That was how Aristotle saw it, in the wisdom of his age: a child is the result of the man's semen retained in the woman's menstrual blood.

St. Thomas Aquinas based his beliefs on the Artistotelian concept that, at some intermediate point, a soul entered the developing fetus—the defining moment when it became a human being. Church doctrine changed over the centuries. Pope Sixtus V ordered severe punishment for abortion in 1588. Three years later, Pope Gregory XIV repealed the ban. Pope Pius IX decreed the Church's present stand, that life begins at conception, in 1869.

In the contemporary Vatican, abortion is roundly condemned, but once again the moment of personhood is at issue. Joseph Cardinal Ratzinger, prefect of the Congregation for the

Doctrine of Faith, declared in 1987 that the Church could not say with any certainty that life, in fact, began at conception. "Most certainly," he said, "no experimental data can be in itself sufficient to force recognition of a spiritual soul." Abortion was a sin, he said, because life *might* begin at conception.

"This declaration expressly leaves aside the question of the moment the spiritual soul is infused," he wrote. "There is not a unanimous tradition. . . . From a moral point of view, this is certain: even if a doubt existed [that] the fruit of conception is already a human being, it is objectively a grave sin to dare to risk murder." In public, the Church simplifies the issue. In its official "declaration" it makes the following prudent statement: "The Magisterium has not expressly committed himself to an affirmation of a philosophic nature." Ultimately, then, Vatican policy is not based on any scientific or metaphysical considerations but on a moral standpoint.

Among Catholics dissension is widespread. In France, a poll reported that more than 50 percent of women surveyed said they were Catholic but would have an abortion. In the United States, the percentage of Catholic women who have had abortions is higher than among women of other religions; this may be because Catholics are hesitant to use effective birth control.

Fundamentalist sects offer a convenient umbrella for anyone's extreme view. Since bringing RU-486 into the world, I have heard them all. None seems to be based on traditional teachings. Even among scientists, some learned minds base extremist views on a personal interpretation of God's design.

In France, a nemesis from the start has been Dr. Jérome Lejeune, medical adviser to the organization Laissez-les Vivre (Let Them Live). In public meetings, he denounced my "human pesticide," blaming me for the potential genocide of billions. Later, I came across a woman who had been his patient. She had a badly deformed child, a victim of Down's syndrome, and was pregnant again. Lejeune recommended that she have the child. If it was also abnormal, he said, it would be a good companion for the other.

His remarks recalled those of that fanatic I once debated on

American television who offered to support my research if I would find a way to arrest spontaneous miscarriages. All potentially deformed children are God's creatures, he argued.

These people are entitled to speak their piece to anyone willing to listen. But their interpretation of science and morality cannot limit the dimensions of a diverse world.

In the absence of scientific or religious definition of when a person begins, there is only the law. An arbitrary, extralegal judgment which stifles a woman's right to a free choice, or which adds another unwanted baby to an overcrowded planet, is as Kuhse and Singer suggest: obscene.

Various legal definitions of viability are good enough. Britain allows abortions on demand up until the twenty-fourth week. France puts the limit at twelve weeks. Either one is scientifically acceptable. I much prefer the French law because it fits with my own perception of human life.

I was happy when Britain reduced the limit from twenty-eight weeks. There is strong medical argument for this: an earlier pregnancy interruption is less harmful to a woman's health. For me, emotion takes hold when a fetus starts to look human. If I can identify a head, an eye, or feet, I can imagine a whole child. This is not science, just personal, human instincts. Most people feel that way. It is why zealots evoke such reaction with photographs of fetuses. And it is why they are distressed that RU-486 acts well before then.

But that is my own view of the beginning of a human life. Others differ. And I am deeply convinced that no one has the right to impose his private sentiment on someone else.

In the continuous process of fetal development, establishing the point at which abortion becomes illegal is an arbitrary act and yet, for societal reasons, a necessary one. Everyone recognizes that even gradual processes can lead to radical transformations. This is as true for the transformation of ice into vapor as for the development of a few embryonic cells into a newborn baby. The notion of colder versus warmer water in a limited temperature range, in fact, may be difficult to perceive and may vary among individuals—our intuitions may tell us there should be a difference, but our perceptions from one person to the next are entirely subjective. If society had to specify legally the point at which cold becomes warm, its decision would be arbitrary. The same is true for abortion. Since medical progress has lowered the limit on the viability of a fetus, I feel that a woman's decision to undergo a voluntary interruption of her pregnancy might be illegal after the twenty-second week. I like the French law with its twelve-week limit, after which the fetus develops with more hormonal autonomy. We should recognize that societal rules governing reproduction are difficult to establish, and we should proceed with the understanding that these rules should be revisable with the advancement of science.

Whatever happens next, RU-486 has gone into the world. More each year, it will contribute to people's lives. To any of us involved, the thrill is untempered by the stir it has caused. For me, it is the *oeuvre* I dreamed of when I observed my artist friends in New York.

Many people believe that while artists create, scientists only discover already existing phenomena. In fact, the processes are much the same. Each researcher has a method, an approach, a style of his own. Intuition moves him as much as knowledge.

An artist stands before a white surface and adds color and form. A scientist looks into a black box—our figurative term for the research elements at hand—and assembles from what is inside. Each creates and discovers. Both are influenced by time and place, and their work corresponds to the society in which they live. Both need inspiration, dedication, persistence, and much work.

Art and science are coming together in vivid form in the forest of Fontainebleau. For fifteen years, Jean Tinguely, Niki de Saint-Phalle, and others have been sculpting an enormous monument. Near a pool which reflects their "blue Klein" (after Yves Klein, the painter they revered), there will be a mobile of the molecule RU-486.

The theologian Mary Hunt in *Conscience* rejects such easily drawn lines as deciding that an individual life starts at fertilization. She focuses on large issues in a fast-changing world. "I suggest that we use justice and not consistency as the hallmark in our ethical life," she writes. "New technologies present new possibilities for which old and hard lines are not necessarily adequate." Indeed, for a moralist or a believer in God, the challenge is formidable. One should attempt to differentiate between what stems from divine revelation and what results from human interpretation and religious tradition. Each generation must redefine its vision of the world and of the Commandments in view of its current understanding of natural phenomena and its social organization. Since scientific knowledge has progressed more dramatically in our generation than ever before in history, the task for us is unprecedented.

It might seem consistent to fix an arbitrary time for the moment when human matter receives the spark of life. But if that rule ends up victimizing women and bringing into the world unwanted children whose lives are doomed from the start, it is not justice. And if those who demand a "right to life" can condemn to death 200,000 women each year, it is not even consistency.

Scientists understand consistency: it is at the heart of what we do. But, more, scientists are human. Justice, in the end, is of higher value.

RU-486 was revealed first to the French Academy of Sciences, to a chilly, even dubious reception. Nearly eight years later, it came back, under the solemn dome across from the Louvre, in the formal annual session. Jean Aubouin, president of the Academy, brought the audience to its feet in thunderous applause with an address on morality and science in the new millennium ahead.

Aubouin, a geologist who looks at mountains and the shifting of the earth's crust, spoke of molecules and the fate of mankind. The pill was his illustration.

People expected Good from science, he said, but science could only offer True. The two are not always the same. It is True that a cat eats mice, but that is only Good to the cat. In the years ahead, society will have to shape Good from the Truths of science.

Aubouin developed his theme: Medicine has added four months to human life for every year of this century. That has brought the world to the brink of potential explosion, a demographic challenge that constitutes its single greatest threat. And medical science hàs addressed that as well, with fertility control. It is no longer necessary to reproduce *en masse* to assure human survival. But demographics are in the hands of society at large.

"The recent controversy around a pill developed by one of our *confrères* shows that a number of [people] refuse to see this," Aubouin said. ". . . Where is the responsibility? Is it with doctors who assure the security of life but also provide the means to limit destructive proliferation? Isn't it rather with those who refuse to take into account new conditions of human life on earth, thus preparing a world of conflict in which the moral values they invoke can only perish?"

Aubouin concluded, "but I believe I am able to predict that all of them lead to the same conclusion: humanity does not suffer from too much science but rather a delay in conceptualizing the world as science has revealed it, and is continuing to reveal it. The dawn of a third millennium demands that we adapt models which have not changed since antiquity, when science was only speculative and the world misunderstood."

Over centuries, our laws and customs have come down from on high, from church or monarchy; the common man was not expected to think for himself. Today, developed societies are increasingly secular. We are able to base our decisions upon scientific discovery. I do not believe that the next century belongs to the fundamentalists or the backward thinkers. Instead, education and science will take us forward, in the directions that we ourselves will choose.

As I listened to Aubouin's address, I reflected on RU-486 and its promise, and the orator's words echoed my own thoughts. In the approaching years, science and the role of women were on the rise. The "abortion pill" would serve both. A new century of light awaits us, Aubouin was saying. "Let us not be afraid."

APPENDIX

RU-486 was originally designated RU-38486, the number of molecules synthesized at Roussel-Uclaf's Romainville laboratories from 1949 to 1980. It is an antiprogesterone, a derivative of norethindrone. The formula is 17β-hydroxy-11β (dimethylaminophenyl)-17α-(1-propynyl)estra-4,9-dien-3-one. Its generic name is mifepristone, and its French trade name is Mifegyne.

When RU-486 was synthesized, Roussel-Uclaf employed three hundred researchers and assistants at Romainville, part of a worldwide staff of fifteen thousand people. Its annual sales were more than 10 billion francs, or about $2 billion.

Hormones and Receptors

"Hormone" comes from the Greek *ormein*, meaning "to excite." Hormones are chemical compounds, information-bearing molecules which act as signals. They are produced by several organs and by the endocrine glands, such as the pituitary at the base of the brain, the thyroid at the front of the neck, the adrenal glands near the kidneys, and the ovaries or the testes.

Hormones are secreted into the bloodstream and, along with oxygen, sugars, and other nutrients, are distributed throughout the body. Their concentration is from 10,000 to 1 million times less than most of the nutritive elements or other components. They are only signal devices, and a very small quantity is needed for their control mission.

A hormone in the bloodstream recognizes only a particular category of cells, the target cells (Figure 1). These alone are able to read the hormonal message; they are equipped with "receptors," as precisely tuned to an individual hormone as a radio must be to a wavelength.

To act, a hormone binds physically, not chemically, to its receptor. As the linkup is temporary, this mechanism is reversible; it is like opening a lock with a key and then withdrawing it, again closing the lock. Once activated, the receptor takes over and transmits the message to the cell. The hormone, after delivering its information, is eliminated by the body. If the function that was triggered is to continue, more hormones must follow to signal more receptors. A higher level of hormones touches many more receptors and intensifies the function; a halt in their supply will stop it.

In the case of progesterone and other steroid hormones of the same chemical category, the receptor is situated in the cen-

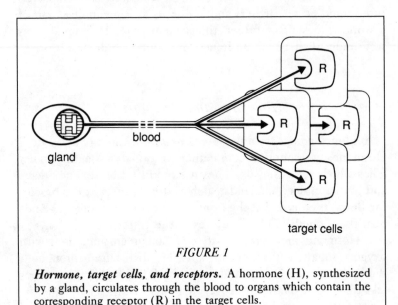

FIGURE 1

Hormone, target cells, and receptors. A hormone (H), synthesized by a gland, circulates through the blood to organs which contain the corresponding receptor (R) in the target cells.

tral part of the cell, the nucleus, where genes are also assembled. The nucleus is surrounded by a membrane, which the hormone must traverse after entering the cell. The receptor is much larger than the hormone molecule. It is a protein, formed by about one thousand amino acids of twenty different structures aligned in a very specific order.

The long chain of amino acids folded within a tridimensional space is a complex structure with several different sectors, or domains, that are crucial to hormonal activity. These were primarily defined by Ron Evans of the Salk Institute in La Jolla, California, and Pierre Chambon in Strasbourg. The first is the LBD, or ligand binding domain (Figure 2). This is like the keyhole. Its structure allows a precise fit for the corresponding hormone. Communication is assured by a number of contact points. Contrary to chemical links, which can rarely be reversed without a powerful outside agent, such binding is undone when contact is broken. Reversibility of hormone action is why the endocrine system is so versatile.

The second sector, the DBD, or DNA binding domain, interacts with the genes to modify their expression. Genes are the chemical basis of heredity, and their transmission during reproduction assures the continuity of a species. Genes are expressed in a unique way in each type of cells, so that muscles, skin, glands, or other organs each function in a particular manner. The regulation of the "genetic expression" in different cells permits a response to needs of the organism.

Unlike hormones and receptors, genes are made up chemically of DNA, rich in phosphoric acid and comprising four variable molecules, the bases. They are aligned specifically, and each group of three signifies one amino acid, according to a code—the "genetic code." This alignment on one of the two tracks of the double helix, shown in Figure 2, determines the structure of each protein made in the cell. Research by James Watson and Francis Crick led to the basic understanding of DNA.

Besides the coding sequences of DNA, there are other segments which have a regulatory role and which modify gene ex-

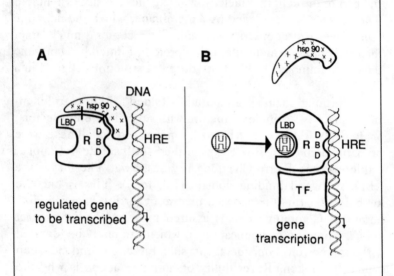

FIGURE 2

Receptor: hormone binding, transformation and activation of genes, role of heat-shock protein. A steroid receptor (R) contains two main domains. One binds with the hormone (H), the ligand binding domain (LBD). The other interacts with DNA, the DNA binding domain (DBD). DNA includes a specific zone for the response to hormones, the hormone response element (HRE), and a template on which ribonucleic acid is formed (indicated by an arrow). In the absence of hormone (A), DBD cannot bind to HRE because it is capped by a heat-shock protein (hsp 90) attached to the receptor. When the hormone binds (B), the receptor's shape changes, which releases the hsp 90. The DBD can then interact with HRE. Additional changes in the receptor (*not shown*) activate gene transcription by an effect on transcription factors (TF).

pression quantitatively. Some, recognized specifically by hormone receptors, are called HREs, hormone response elements. Interaction with HREs is necessary to modify the functioning of the genes, probably by reorganizing the complex arrangement called chromatin. Besides DNA, chromatin involves many proteins influencing gene function.

Other sectors of the receptor, called transcriptional activators, can interact with other proteins, such as transcription factors (TF), which themselves act at the DNA level to modify gene expression. Hormone binding activates the interplay between receptors and TF.

In sum, the LBD part of the receptor receives the hormonal message which changes its shape. The other parts, the DBD and activators, then provoke the hormonal response at the gene level. In its inactive state, the LBD is capped by a "heat-shock protein," hsp 90 (90,000 molecular weight). This was demonstrated in my laboratory, particularly by Maria-Grazia Catelli and Jan Mester, and with the help of James Feramisco and William Welsh, of the Cold Spring Harbor Laboratory in New York. When the LBD is activated by a hormone, it throws off the hsp 90 cap, and the receptor physically entwines with the double helix of DNA (Figure 2B).

The word "steroid" designates a chemical structure related to cholesterol. Cholesterol, abundant in the body, is part of all membranes that surround the cells and delimit the nucleus and other compartments. Some of it circulates in the blood and comes partly from the liver, which synthesizes it, and partly from food, after intestinal absorption. Along with its part in forming membranes, cholesterol produces several important compounds, including steroid hormones.

To make these, cholesterol enters in appreciable quantities into the cells of the adrenal glands, ovaries, testes, and, during pregnancy, the placenta, which temporarily functions as an endocrine gland. In these glandular cells, cholesterol is modified chemically, while keeping its basic steroid structure, to form hormones which will be secreted.

Steroid hormones, produced from a part of the initial cholesterol molecule, are about two hundred times smaller than their receptors. They are lipidic (fatty) molecules—unlike proteins, which are more soluble in water—and easily penetrate cellular membranes, which are themselves mostly formed of lipids. Steroid properties differ, depending upon their detailed chemical structure. Corticosteroids mainly affect metabolism while sex steroids act mostly upon reproductive organs.

Progesterone

Progesterone, chemically speaking, is relatively simple. Its atoms form a flat ensemble (Figure 3A). It is a steroid with fewer chemical groups than cortisol, the adrenal hormone with the properties of cortisone. Cortisol does not bind to the progesterone receptor. But progesterone, smaller, binds to the receptor of glucocorticosteroids.

Progesterone was first isolated in 1929 at the University of Rochester by George Corner and Willard Allen, within ovaries of the sow. Injected into test animals, it spectacularly altered the endometrium, which makes up the lining of the uterus, where the embryo implants. In 1910, Paul Ancel and Paul Bouin in France had watched this change in rabbits; they called it "uterine lace." The transformation, caused by progesterone, allows implantation.

Further studies showed that progesterone was essential to maintaining pregnancy. Without it, or a progestin, which is a different compound with similar biological properties (an analog), the mother miscarried. Progesterone is secreted after midcycle by the corpus luteum in the ovary, which forms after the follicle ruptures to release the egg (Figures 4 and 5).

The corpus luteum gives its name to the second part of the menstrual cycle, the luteal phase. Along with preparing the endometrium for implantation, progesterone does two things which help prevent expulsion of the blastocyst: it relaxes contractions of the myometrium, the muscle forming the womb, and tightens

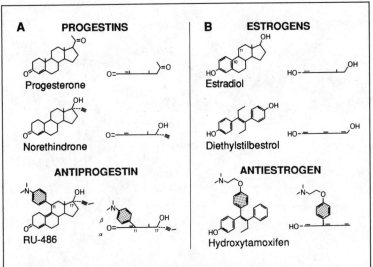

A   PROGESTINS

Progesterone

Norethindrone

ANTIPROGESTIN

RU-486

B   ESTROGENS

Estradiol

Diethylstilbestrol

ANTIESTROGEN

Hydroxytamoxifen

FIGURE 3

Chemical formulas of natural hormones, synthetic analogues, and antihormones. Molecule structures are shown in polycyclic form, face, and profile. Figure 3A shows progestins and the antiprogestin RU-486. Figure 3B shows estrogens and the antiestrogen hydroxytamoxifen.

A. Progesterone is a natural hormone, and norethindrone is a synthetic analog, which was used in the first contraceptive pills. RU-486 differs from norethindrone in the cycle grafted from the carbon 11 atom (shaded) and another group on the carbon 17 atom. The prominent cycle branched on carbon 11 can be seen in profile.

B. Estradiol is a natural estrogen, and diethylstilbestrol is a synthetic compound which has lost part of the steroid structure but is still a potent estrogen. Hydroxytamoxifen is a synthetic antiestrogen, different from diethylstilbestrol because of a grafted cycle (shaded) which resembles that which distinguishes RU-486 from norethin-·drone.

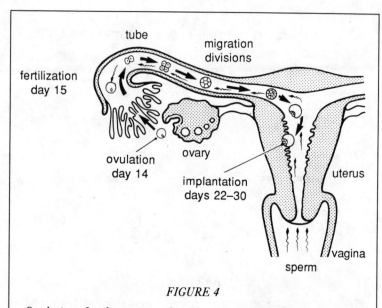

FIGURE 4

Ovulation, fertilization, and implantation. After fertilization, the zygote migrates toward the uterus as it divides and develops into an embryo. At about day 22, called a blastocyst because of its tiny cavity, it starts to implant in the uterine wall.

the cervix, the opening of the uterus in the vagina. Conversely, at childbirth, progesterone flow stops, permitting the necessary contractions and dilation of the cervix.

In the absence of implantation, there is luteolysis, the destruction of the corpus luteum. Progesterone diminishes (Figure 5A), and cells of the transformed endometrium die away. This produces menstruation, made up of blood and cellular debris. If there is implantation, the blastocyst triggers a new control of progesterone secretion. Its cells form an annex, the chorion, to the developing embryo core which secretes a nonsteroidal hormone called chorionic gonadotropin, or hCG (human chorionic gonadotropin).

Implantation (Figures 4, 6A, and 6B) gives hCG access to

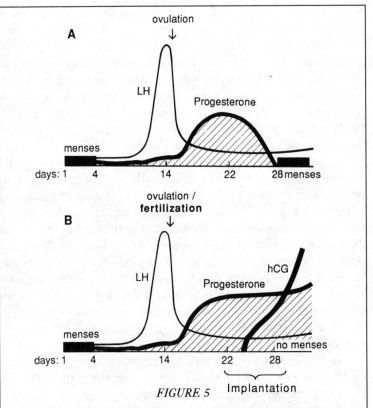

FIGURE 5 Implantation

Hormones during a nonfertile cycle and at the beginning of pregnancy.

A. During a 28-day nonfertile cycle, the peak of luteinizing hormone (LH) triggers ovulation, and the corpus luteum secretes progesterone. When the corpus luteum decays, progesterone decreases and menses occurs.

B. After implantation hCG enters the woman's body and sustains the corpus luteum, which secretes larger amounts of progesterone. There is no menses.

(Curves show the change in hormone concentration in the blood in arbitrary units. The well-known pattern in temperature increase during the second part of the cycle and the beginning of pregnancy, and that of progesterone concentration in the blood, are almost superimposable.)

the maternal organs, passing via blood vessels of the uterus. A pregnancy test is based on detecting in blood or urine this hormone emanating from the embryo. Mainly, hCG stimulates the corpus luteum, preventing it from regressing as during a nonfertile cycle. Thus affected, menstrual corpus luteum becomes gravidic corpus luteum, which secretes increased levels of progesterone. This signals the lower brain and pituitary gland to block the secretion of luteinizing hormone (LH) and prevents the release of another egg during pregnancy.

After eight to ten weeks, hCG diminishes progressively, and the corpus luteum regresses along with it. The placenta, now well developed next to the embryo, takes charge of producing progesterone itself. This is necessary to control the function of the uterine lining and the myometrium until delivery. Hormone distribution is now changed (Figure 6C). The placenta is in contact with the uterus, the target of progesterone. Part of the hormone is also secreted directly to the developing embryo, now a fetus. It plays no direct part in fetal development but it converts partially into other hormones, such as corticosteroids.

At childbirth, the drop in progesterone permits the muscle fibers of the myometrium to respond to oxytocic agents, such as prostaglandin and oxytocin, which provoke contractions. Oxytocin is a hormone secreted from the posterior part of the pituitary. It is sometimes administered to ease delivery. Also, the decrease in progesterone allows the production of milk, which the hormone blocked during pregnancy.

RU-486 is meant to oppose the effect of progesterone in preparing for and sustaining pregnancy. However, other biological aspects of progesterone are relevant to the possible effects of the compound.

During the female cycle, we have seen that progesterone intervenes after ovulation, during the luteal phase, but it also has an earlier role. The luteinizing hormone, secreted from the anterior part of the pituitary gland, is chemically and functionally similar to the placental hCG which takes over to stop the corpus luteum from regressing in pregnancy. The peak point of LH secretion

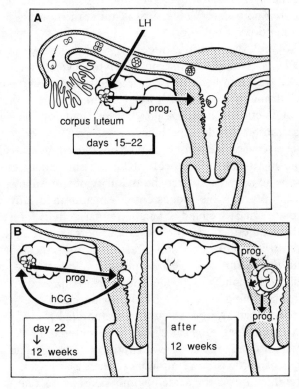

FIGURE 6

Three periods after fertilization. A. During migration and division of the developing embryo, for one week, the pituitary hormone LH stimulates the corpus luteum to make progesterone, which prepares the endometrium for implantation.

B. During the following weeks, implantation is completed and progesterone is needed for maintaining the endometrium, which has become the decidua. The hormone made at the base (chorion) of the embryo, human chorionic gonadotropin (hCG), enters the mother's blood and stimulates progesterone secretion by the corpus luteum. A pregnancy test detects the presence of hCG.

C. After 12 weeks, the corpus luteum is no longer needed to secrete progesterone; the placenta, an annex of the embryo as it is becoming a fetus, serves this purpose until delivery.

during the cycle occurs by day 14 and triggers ovulation, about twenty-four hours later. This burst is under the double control of estradiol and progesterone.

Estradiol, the natural estrogen, is synthesized by the ovarian follicle cells during the first phase of the cycle, the follicular phase. At the end of this phase, these cells also produce progesterone, although at a much lower level than during the luteal phase. A fraction is secreted just before ovulation, and a small increase can be found in the blood (Figure 5A). As faint as it is, this increase of progesterone could nonetheless have an important role in triggering the peak of LH. Also, part of this early progesterone seems to affect the maturity of the follicle and its point of rupture. This progesterone remains in the ovary and could have what is called a parahormonal activity. That is, it might have an effect near the location of hormonal production as opposed to its normal function of acting at a distance after travelling in the blood. These early progesterone activities imply a potential to respond to RU-486 before ovulation.

Besides being produced by the ovaries and the placenta, progesterone can also be isolated in the adrenal glands. But except in certain pathological cases, it is secreted in very small amounts into the blood; it is an intermediate product of the synthesis of corticosteroid hormones, such as cortisol. In other words, although it is the same chemical product as that made in other glands, adrenal progesterone is not a hormone. It is not addressed to a receptor. And it has no other role than that of a precursor product, and RU-486 does not affect it.

These examples show that the same compound that is formed at different points in time or by different cells might not have the same function or significance in the body. The chemistry of a molecule is not enough to define it physiologically. Biological analysis of a given molecule's function should take into account not only chemistry but also the anatomical arrangement of the body and sequences of events.

Progesterone target cells are found classically in the reproductive organs: the uterus, the fallopian tubes, the vagina, the pituitary gland and the hypothalamus, the ovaries, and the mammary glands. The activity of these organs is partly coordinated by progesterone in reproduction. Beyond the zones of the hypothalamus, controlling the pituitary gland, we also have found progesterone receptors elsewhere in the nervous system. If these receptors are accessible to the hormone, they might also be accessible to a corresponding antihormone, which could be medically important.

Although hormones of each sex—androgens in the man and estrogens in the woman—are found in small quantities in the other, almost no progesterone circulates in the male bloodstream. Nonetheless, it is possible that, as in animals, small quantities are synthesized in the central nervous system of both sexes, probably for local activity.

RU-486, An Antiprogesterone

Any method that can counter the effect of a hormone is called antihormonal. Several means allow this, at least in principle.

One can envisage suppressing the biosynthesis of the hormone: it would disappear, its effects with it. Epostane, a steroid derivative, blocks the formation of progesterone in the corpus luteum and placenta. But it can equally suppress this biosynthesis in the adrenal glands and, as a result, deprive the body of cortisol, which can be detrimental.

It would seem theoretically possible to intercept progesterone on its way toward the uterine target. This can be done experimentally with animals, using an antiprogesterone antibody, as demonstrated by Brian Heap in Cambridge (England). The principle, however, seems impossible to apply to women. It is likewise difficult to use a method that would selectively deactivate a circulating hormone by a metabolic mechanism.

The place where we can be certain the progesterone is recognized, and where it sets off a hormonal response, is the receptor. Action at this point is specific and immediate, and interacting there, an antihormone blocks the transmission of the hormone's message. This is the function of RU-486.

The compound has a basic steroid structure (see Figure 3A). In certain details, its structure compares closely with that of norethindrone, a synthesized progestin which remains very active when taken orally and for this reason was used in an oral contraceptive pill in the early 1960s. Progesterone itself is rendered largely inactive if it passes through the intestines and liver after ingestion. What chemically characterizes RU-486 is the important supplementary nucleus (a dimethylaminophenyl group) grafted on the number 11 carbon atom and pointing to the upper side of the plane of the molecule. This forms an appendage which is principally responsible for antiprogesterone activity.

Specialized publications now provide a long list of chemical derivatives, often close to RU-486, which have since been synthesized by chemists at Roussel-Uclaf, Schering in Germany, Organon in the Netherlands, and other companies.

It is remarkable that the graft of a voluminous chemical grouping on the fairly flat form of a steroid does not preclude high affinity binding to a receptor. One would suppose that the niche of the LBD receptor requires a tight fit of the natural hormone so that the interaction is specific. But it would have to be sufficiently supple to adapt to a molecule of quite a different form, or present an additional cavity that is not used with a natural steroid but is able to accommodate the extra group. The same observation would apply to the other chemical sequence added to the number 17 carbon atom (see Figure 3A), even though it is much smaller.

A structural reshuffling must take place in the receptor molecule, touched off by the impact of RU-486. One of the results is that the receptor holds more tightly to the hsp 90 protein, the opposite of what happens when an active hormone binds to the receptor. The hormone is an agonist, an agent that acts positively. The antihormone is an antagonist; it tends to prevent the hsp 90 protein from separating to pass on a hormonal message to the DNA. However, the molecular mechanism is more complex; the stabilization of hsp 90 is itself reversible, and very likely the receptor is so deformed that activation of the transcription factor does not occur (Figure 7). In molecular terms, much remains unknown to scientists.

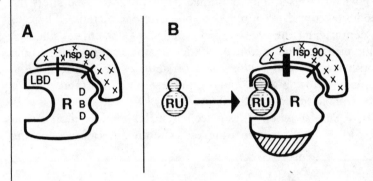

FIGURE 7

Progesterone receptor and RU-486. A. In the absence of binding by RU-486, the progesterone receptor is identical to that shown in Figure 2A.

B. After binding by RU-486, two changes in the receptor are shown here. The hsp 90 cap is not released as when a hormone binds to the receptor; instead, it binds more tightly. Also, a change in the receptor form (shaded area) indicates that it might have a role in modifying the transcription factor function (see Figure 2B).

Whatever the details, the basic workings are clear. When RU-486 is administered, it competes with progesterone to bind to the receptor. The result depends on the concentration of the two steroids. The less progesterone there is to neutralize, the greater the effectiveness of RU-486, and conversely. The compound has essentially no other direct effect of its own.

Gary Hodgen, at NIH and the Jones Foundation laboratories, made studies of antihormonal effects on spayed monkeys. The ovaries were removed, and an artificial cycle was established by administering estradiol and progesterone at their natural levels. The uterus was then prepared for implantation, as during the luteal phase. Administering RU-486 provoked menstrual bleeding within forty-eight hours. The controlled presence of progesterone proved that RU-486 was an effective antagonist.

These experiments allow an understanding of how the antihormone can interrupt pregnancy in an animal or a woman.

Progesterone is still at its normal level when RU-486 alters the
endometrium by suppressing progesterone action. There is
bleeding, and the embryo and its annexes detach, causing as a
side effect a drop in human chorionic gonadotropin going to the
mother (Figure 8). This, in turn, reduces stimulation of the
gravidic corpus luteum, and less progesterone is secreted. This is
a secondary effect of RU-486.

A similar action takes place when RU-486 interrupts a nonfertile cycle. By suppressing progesterone, it causes bleeding

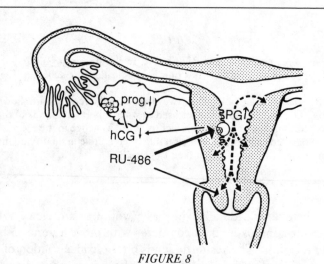

FIGURE 8

**Primary and secondary effects of RU-486 at the beginning of preg-
nancy.** The main effect of RU-486 is to block progesterone action in
the endometrium and then provoke alteration of implantation with
bleeding. There is also a direct activity on the cervix, which is soft-
ened and opened.

Secondary effects are of two categories. One is increased prostaglandin concentration in the altered endometrium. Prostaglandin
stimulates contractility of the myometrium, the muscle of the uterus
(Figure 9), and also softens and opens the cervix. In the other, the
detachment of the embryo leads to a decrease in hCG; the corpus
luteum is no longer stimulated and progesterone secretion diminishes. As a result, the embryo is expelled with bleeding, and the
ovarian function returns to normal.

from the endometrium and a secondary regression of the corpus luteum, with the subsequent effect of permitting the synthesis of luteinizing hormone (LH), which signals the release of an egg for the next cycle.

Prostaglandins

Prostaglandins—shortened to PG, followed by letters and numbers to designate their variety—play many important roles in the body. They are structurally different from steroids. They form a category of local-action hormones synthesized from certain "polyunsaturated" fatty acids. Polyunsaturated fatty acids have several double bonds, which make them more chemically unstable than ordinary fats, which are saturated by hydrogen and resemble paraffin. These fatty acids, constituting vitamin F ("F" for fat), are not made by the body but are indispensable to health. These are essential to diet precisely because they are the precursors of prostaglandins.

The synthesis of prostaglandins involves the formation of a cycle by part of the fatty acid molecule. This very complex process can be blocked by anti-inflammatory medicines, like aspirin, as observed by John Vane in England. Studies of prostaglandins during the 1960s and 1970s, particularly by Sune Bergström and Bengt Samuelsson in Sweden, help explain a number of phenomenona in physiology, pharmacology, and pathology.

Among the most important activities of prostaglandins is their stimulation of smooth muscle fibers. Along with the body's skeletal muscles are "smooth" muscles, of a different nature, which respond to different stimuli. They ensure the mobility of the stomach and intestines and the tone of blood vessels. The myometrium is smooth muscle. An injection of prostaglandin can provoke contractions of the uterus, but also the muscles of the digestive tract and the heart.

During an abortion with RU-486, the level of prostaglandins increases in the uterus. They can be measured in the uterus or the blood, as originally seen in observations by Walter Herrmann in Geneva. This is probably because of tissue alteration which occurs after RU-486 has suppressed the progesterone effect on the endometrium (Figure 8). Bernard Descomps in Montpellier showed that RU-486 inhibits the release of a prostaglandin derivative, prostacycline (PGI_2), which relaxes the tension of muscle fibers. This complementary effect of RU-486 may contribute to augmenting the contractions of the myometrium.

An increase in prostaglandins also accompanies a normal birth. They play an important physiological part, as oxytocic agents stimulating the uterus and are responsible for the painful contractions. In addition, prostaglandins themselves directly dilate and soften the cervix.

During an abortion, the phenomena are similar but less intense. The detachment of the embryo, because of the antiprogesterone effect, leads to an increase in the concentration of prostaglandins, which heighten contractions of the myometrium. Moreover, prostaglandins soften the cervical opening, facilitating expulsion. The increase of prostaglandins has mostly a local effect, with only a limited diffusion throughout the body, where they would cause secondary digestive reactions.

Thus, there are two successive phases during abortion by RU-486. First, its direct action on the endometrium, with subsequent bleeding which carries away the detached embryo, leads to a decrease in hCG and an increase in prostaglandins. Second, there are contractions of the myometrium, the opening of the cervix, and a drop in the production of progesterone.

Clinical Testing of RU-486 Only

The first trials for abortion by RU-486 were done at the Department of Reproduction at Cantonal Hospital in Geneva, directed by Dr. Walter Herrmann, after clearance by toxicologists and the local ethics committee. The patients, all volunteers, had amenorrhea of six to eight weeks' duration. (Amenorrhea, meaning the absence of menstrual bleeding, is counted from the first day of the last period.)

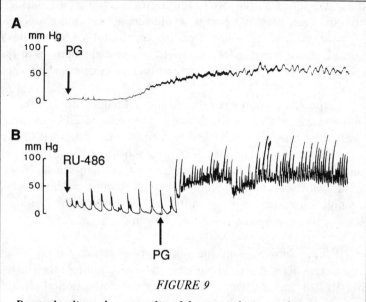

FIGURE 9

Prostaglandin and contractility of the uterus during early pregnancy.
This graph shows the contractions of the uterus in a woman with a
pregnancy of about 10 weeks, as recorded by Drs. M. Bygdeman and
M. I. Swahn of the Karolinska Hospital in Stockholm.

A. Contractions are few in the absence of any treatment, but they
intensify with the administration of prostaglandin in a dose insufficient to induce abortion.

B. RU-486 alone triggers contractions, which increase substantially
with the addition of the same small dose of prostaglandin.

(Curves indicate the pressure developed by uterine contractions
expressed in millimeters of mercury.)

Typically, fertilization occurs on the fifteenth day of a cycle,
or two weeks after the start of the last period. Implantation
begins on the twenty-second day. It is completed during the
fourth week of the cycle, to the twenty-eighth day. A late period
suggests possible pregnancy, which can be diagnosed rapidly by
measuring hCG in the blood. The test is based on the immunological reaction of a part of the molecule.

Each woman received a total of 200 mg of RU-486 a day for

four days, administered two or four times daily in 50-mg pills. In a typical case, bleeding began on the second day and expulsion followed on the fourth day. Bleeding continued for several days more. Uterine cramps, felt mainly until' the expulsion, were relieved by an analgesic. Progesterone and hCG diminished after expulsion.

Later trials conducted by André Ulmann and Catherine Dubois were with a single dose of three pills of 200 mg each, taken all at once. This method was equally effective, since the compound has a relatively slow metabolism: its half-life—the time that it takes for half of it to be destroyed in the body—is about twenty-four hours, much longer than most hormones. A single dose was an important simplification of the method. Results were less satisfactory with a single dose of under 600 mg.

Taking into account the obligatory seven-day wait under French law, RU-486 could not be administered before the thirty-fifth day of amenorrhea, a week after the day a period should have started. RU-486 taken in a single 600-mg dose within forty-two days of amenorrhea showed results of about 80 percent effectiveness. Expulsion was complete after three to five days, and bleeding stopped within an average of ten days. Total blood volume, measured in British testing, averaged 90 ml, the same as heavy menstruation. It was recommended not to take aspirin or any other post-steroid anti-inflammatory drug which can decrease production of prostaglandin in the body.

In case of failure, aspiration or curettage was necessary. This was because of excessive bleeding or because of remaining tissue, which could have caused a secondary infection. When pregnancy continued, in 1 percent of the cases, bleeding was minimal or nonexistent and a surgical abortion was performed.

Abortion with RU-486 and a Prostaglandin

The use of 600 mg of RU-486 followed two days later by a small dose of prostaglandin (Figure 10) brought the effectiveness rate to 95 percent or higher. The process simply complemented the natural production of prostaglandin in the uterus. Progesterone is neutralized by RU-486 and cannot calm the effects of prostaglandins. As a result, a small amount is extremely active in the uterus (see Figure 9) but not in the digestive tract or the vascular system.

An abortion can be induced with prostaglandins alone, but the dosage must be very high to counteract progesterone. This stimulates all of the body's smooth muscles, provoking nausea, vomiting, diarrhea, and sometimes changes in arterial pressure and even cardiac function. With a small dose given to supplement RU-486, these side effects are minimized.

By 1991, the effectiveness rate in France after more than 70,000 cases was about 95 percent, the same as the early tests conducted in Sweden, England, China, Hungary, Spain, Holland, Italy, and Singapore. In France, the method may be used up to the forty-ninth day of amenorrhea. Tests in Britain showed identical results when used at sixty-three days, or five weeks after a missed period should have begun.

In 5 percent of cases, the embryo is expelled within two days, and a prostaglandin is not necessary. In France, for reasons of cost and availability, clinics mostly prescribed an injection of 0.25 or 0.5 mg of sulprostone, a derivative of PGE_2, sold as Nalador by Schering, Berlin. In some cases, they used a vaginal suppository of prostaglandin of another chemical type, 1 mg of gemeprost, a derivative of PGE_1, marketed as Cervagen. Other prostaglandins are under study, including the very active meteneprost (a PGE_2 analogue).

In 1991, Dr. Elisabeth Aubény and I conducted trials in Paris with misoprostol, a PGE_1 derivative, which is taken orally. The 400-microgram dose was half the normal daily amount prescribed for the treatment of gastroduodenal ulcer patients. The effectiveness rate was slightly higher than that of sulprostone and gemeprost. Women reported only mild cramps.

The making of a single pill, containing RU-486 and time-released prostaglandin, is under study.

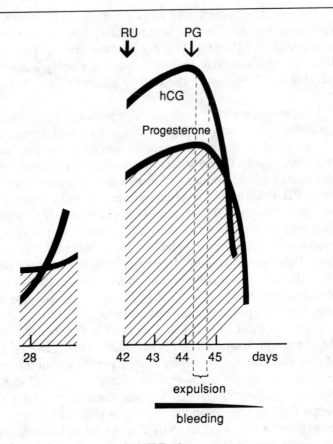

FIGURE 10

Six-week pregnancy interruption with RU-486. The curves follow those of Figure 5. At six weeks of pregnancy, progesterone and hCG have augmented. RU-486 (600 mg) is given at this point, along with prostaglandin (PG) two days later. Expulsion follows, with a rapid decrease of hCG and progesterone. Bleeding which preceded expulsion stops in a few days.

(Curves indicate the change of concentration of hormones in the blood in arbitrary units; see also Figure 5B.)

Fetotoxicity

Fetotoxicity refers to the risk of damage to the fetus in case of a failure of RU-486 with no follow-up instrumental extraction. This is difficult to study because the fetus is expelled with a high dose of RU-486, and it is not exposed to prolonged use. RU-486 works at the level of the endometrium and the myometrium; abortion results from action on the uterus, not the fetus. However, if pregnancy is not terminated, as occurs in about 1 percent of cases, possible repercussions must be considered.

Alfred Jost at the Collège de France showed in studies with rabbits that if the ovaries are removed during pregnancy, the animal needs a certain dose of progesterone to continue a normal pregnancy. Without progesterone, it aborts. If intermediate doses are administered, the uterus contracts abnormally and causes lesions of the skull and central nervous system of the fetus. In rabbits with ovaries intact, RU-486 administered in doses of less than that required for an abortion provokes lesions identical with those caused by progesterone insufficiency in spayed rabbits.

This muscular activity in the uterus seems to be specific to rabbits. Similar fetal anomalies could not be reproduced in rats or guinea pigs. Also, Jost's experiments were with pregnancies that were far more advanced than those treated with RU-486. Nonetheless, the results suggest that instrumental evacuation should be used when RU-486 does not terminate pregnancy.

To complete the tests and determine any possible fetotoxicity of RU-486, the compound was given to animals in high doses at different stages of pregnancy, from the beginning to the end. Progesterone was given to counteract the antiprogesterone effect in order to observe any toxicity independent of the abortive action. Nothing abnormal was noted in any of the cases, including the case of the small monkeys which were followed for several years in Gary Hodgen's laboratory. Extrapolation of animal results to humans is always somewhat arbitrary, which is another reason to recommend instrumental abortion in the case of RU-486 failure.

Using RU-486 to facilitate delivery poses a serious problem, that of ensuring the future health of the child, particularly because RU-486 passes into the fetus. Scientific logic, especially the reversible effect and specific target of RU-486, excludes a priori any danger to the baby. But it seems as if the use of RU-486 in such cases should be restricted to life-threatening situations. It is difficult to decide between the certain advantages of a method and its possible complications. Any choice, in medicine, is seldom without risk.

Genotoxicity

Here the risk is toxicity at the most fundamental level, the genes, which might be affected during the very early stages of the embryo. For biological reasons related to the action of hormones, there is little chance that any anomaly would develop. Experiments were performed dealing with fertilization in test tubes. Gary Hodgen exposed monkey embryos to high levels of RU-486. After reimplantation in the uterus, the embryos showed normal development, confirming other studies on a number of different species. Nonetheless, prudence suggests that further studies should be done.

Along with the theoretical and experimental evidence, there were three cases in Britain and two in France where women decided to continue their pregnancies after RU-486 failed. All five babies were normal.

Antiglucocorticosteroid Activity

Cortisol is a hormone of the adrenal glands which is essential in the body's adaptation to stress. It alters the metabolism of sugars, fats and proteins, and is involved in immunological and blood pressure regulation, as well as several brain functions. The drop in prostaglandins that it triggers partly explains the anti-inflammatory effect of corticosteroids like cortisone and synthetic analogues used in therapy.

RU-486 is the first antiglucocorticosteroid active in humans, and it is very efficient in treating certain tumors associated with Cushing's syndrome. It has a great affinity for the glucocorticosteroid receptor. Since RU-486 opposes the effects of cortisol, it can be suspected of provoking an acute adrenal insufficiency in healthy people. This was observed in giving very high doses to animals.

Logic and evidence alleviate these concerns when RU-486 is used for abortion, except in cases of patients already suffering from adrenal insufficiency. Cortisol is part of a well-integrated endocrine network, under the control of hypothalamic and pituitary hormones which stimulate its production in the case of insufficiency. A dose of 200 mg or more of RU-486 in an adult provokes an antiglucocorticosteroid effect by blocking the receptor, but this causes the body to counterbalance the loss with an increase of cortisol.

This explains a temporary adrenal reaction which stops after administration of RU-486. Thus, there is no hypotension, drop in glycemia, or other effects, as might have been feared.

A prolonged use of RU-486, in treating certain cancers or other pathological conditions, will require new toxicology and tolerance tests. These tests would depend upon the dosage and the timing of administration. Probably other antiprogesterones will be discovered with antiprogesterone and antiglucocorticosteroid activities of RU-486, dissociated from one another. Roussel-Uclaf chemists are working on these for the future.

Toxicity and Side Effects

The first tests of RU-486 were performed on rats and monkeys before use in humans. The tests showed a remarkable tolerance for RU-486. It produced no anomaly, neither functionally nor biochemically, in the liver, kidneys, cardiovascular system, blood chemistry, nervous system, or other organs. Tests were conducted with doses far higher than those necessary for abortion.

Scientists know that any biologically active product may have side effects under special circumstances which occur with long use. This has been the case with aspirin, penicillin, and vaccines. As a result, post-marketing surveillance and further research continue and should never stop. However, as a steroid, RU-486 leaves the body within several days, leaving behind no trace. It is, as the Americans put it, particularly "clean." As with other well-tested drugs, we can be prudently optimistic.

ACKNOWLEDGMENTS

I WOULD LIKE TO THANK those who have helped me in writing this book, by giving me documents, opinions, editing, etc.: Yvette Akwa, Anne Atger, Yolande Baulieu, Sylviane Bellorini, Catherine Blair, Dr. Rod Bretherton, Professor Marc Bygdeman, Françoise Cachin, Dr. Maria-Grazia Catelli, Professor Rebecca Cook, Professor Georges David, Dr. Henry David, Professor Egon Diczfalusy, Dr. Catherine Euvrard, Jean-Luc Fidel, Father Norman Ford, Joan Furlong, Dr. Bernard Gore, Simone Harari, Professor Walter Herrmann, Professor Gary Hodgen, Dr. Sven Lindenberg, Victoria Mancuso, Senator Elena Marinucci, Ariel Mouttet, Brigitte Ouvry-Vial, Dr. Daniel Philibert, Dr. Malcolm Potts, Dr. Alexandre Psychoyos, Dr. Paul Robel, Niki de Saint-Phalle, Dr. Michaël Schumacher, Professor Roger Short, Professor Claude Sureau, Dr. Georges Teutsch, Adrienne Thievent, Gabrielle Van Zuylen, Jo Wainer, Faye Wattleton, and Professor Samuel Yen.

I am grateful to Françoise Boussac, Philippe Leclerc, Corinne Legris, Father Norman Ford, and Claude Secco, who assisted me in producing the manuscript; and Jean-Claude Lambert, who drew the figures.

I also want to acknowledge the assistance of my editor, Marie Arana-Ward, the enthusiasm of my agent, Irving Lazar, and, last but not least, the remarkable talent of Mort Rosenblum.

This book could never have been written without my great entourage of research companions over the years.

The "Abortion Pill" is adapted from *Génération Pilule*, published in June 1990 by Editions Odile Jacob. It has been updated and recast for an English-speaking readership. The original French version includes more specific scientific data and appropriate references to biomedical journals, which may interest professionals and students.

INDEX